THE

A L L E R G Y
SOURCEBOOK

THE
ALLERGY SOURCEBOOK

EVERYTHING YOU NEED TO KNOW

MERLA ZELLERBACH

FOREWORD BY VINCENT A. MARINKOVICH, M.D.

Lowell House
Los Angeles

Contemporary Books
Chicago

Library of Congress Cataloging-in-Publication Data
Zellerbach, Merla.
  The allergy sourcebook : everything you need to know / by Merla
Zellerbach : foreword by Vincent A. Marinkovich.
    p.   cm.
  Includes index.
  ISBN 1-56565-208-8
  1. Allergy—Popular works.   I. Title.
  RC584.Z45   1995
  616.97—dc20   94-43948
                                                   CIP

Requests for such permissions should be addressed to:
Lowell House
2029 Century Park East, Suite 3290
Los Angeles, CA 90067

Lowell House books can be purchased at special discounts when ordered in bulk for premiums and special sales. Contact Department VH at the address above.

Publisher: Jack Artenstein
General Manager/Editor-in-Chief: Bud Sperry
Text Design: Electric Dragon Productions / Kate Mueller

Manufactured in the United States of America
10 9 8 7 6 5 4 3 2

ALSO BY MERLA ZELLERBACH

Love in a Dark House
Type 1/Type 2 Allergy Relief Program (with Alan Levin, M.D.)
Detox (with Phyllis Saifer, M.D., M.P.H.)
The Wildes of Nob Hill
Love the Giver
Cavett Manor
Sugar
Rittenhouse Square

To Laura and Randy:
May you grow up in a cleaner, healthier world.

CONTENTS

PART IV — ASTHMA 109

PART V — MULTIPLE CHEMICAL SENSITIVITY
(Environmental Illness) 137

PART VI — HELP YOURSELF TO HEALTH 177

APPENDICES

ACKNOWLEDGMENTS

My special thanks to members of the medical profession who shared their time and expertise: Dr. Sheldon Cohen (National Institute of Allergy and Infectious Diseases), Dr. James Davis, Dr. John H. Epstein, Dr. Alan Levin, Dr. Jerome Oremland, Dr. Ben Robinson and his wife, Gloria, Dr. Ernest Rosenbaum and his wife, Izzy, Dr. Edward O'Connell (Mayo School of Medicine), Dr. Martin Valentine (Johns Hopkins University), and especially Dr. Vincent A. Marinkovich who took great pains to keep me up-to-date and accurate.

Grateful mention to Major Richard Haines, Clyde Thom, Janice Gallagher, who inspired me to write this book, and her husband, Derek; Janet McDonald, Susie Sensabaugh, and Michael Hooton of the FDA; Planetree Health Resource Center; The National Jewish Center for Immunology and Respiratory Medicine; Mary Lamielle of the National Center for Environmental Health Strategies.

Added gratitude for editing help to dear friends Ann and Dr. Bob Seymour, to Lee Munson, and to Susan Springer of the Environmental Health Network.

Love and thanks to my children, Linda and Gary Zellerbach, to my sister, Dev Kettner, for crab cakes and moral support, to my sister-in-law Elizabeth Burstein, and to my brother, Dr. Sandor Burstein, for medical literature, advice, and being able to spot a misplaced comma at fifty paces.

Last and far from least, the book owes its existence to the patience of my agent, Fred Hill, my editor, Bud Sperry, and the encouragement and forbearing of my beloved late husband, Fred Goerner.

FOREWORD

Knowledge about and treatment of allergy have come a long way in recent years, but there's still a distance to go.

Symptoms of traditional allergy, such as a runny nose, fits of sneezing, tearing eyes, and itchy skin, are now known to be caused by a specific antibody called IgE, a protein molecule the body produces to fight off foreign substances.

The traditional allergist chooses to focus his attention on IgE-mediated diseases because this is what he was trained to do, and this is what his preferred method of testing, the skin test, can detect. While many people are helped by traditional methods, others are not. Persons with immunological non-IgE-mediated illnesses often have no place to go for diagnosis and treatment.

Adverse reactions to foods, for instance, will get patients referred to gastroenterologists, many of whom do not believe in food allergy; migraine headaches are treated by neurologists who have no training in immunology; joint stiffness/ swelling/ pain is handled by rheumatologists who largely deny any environmental cause for the problems; chronic sinus disease is treated by the ear-nose-throat specialist whose training is drug-oriented and surgical. For all these patients, the treatment will almost certainly be aimed at symptoms, not causes.

At the same time, these patients are exposed to varied and conflicting opinions and have no way to know what is appropriate for them. There is a small cadre of physicians who do try to help. Most are trained as allergists or have some allergy training and experience. They believe in environmental causes of disease and search for them among their patients. They also theorize that non-IgE allergy exists.

Their methods, however, sometimes appear to be at the cutting edge of science (or fringe, if one is being critical) and lack the double-blind clinical studies that traditionalists demand. It is surprising how often double-blind studies published in reputable journals *do* support a method, yet the specialist will remain skeptical to the point of denial and inaction. The phrase, "I haven't seen a proper study" is used to mean that, therefore, such a method or theory is wrong. The intelligent, thoughtful, disabled patient is left with no place to turn.

This book will help fill the information gap. It discusses controversial and sensitive issues with an educated, commonsense authority that was clearly developed from much investigation and many interviews with physicians. It will be widely read by the vast numbers of patients with symptoms suggestive of allergy—those helped by traditional medicine as well as those for whom traditional medicine has not provided answers. The author is to be commended for her excellent handling of a most difficult and complex subject.

Vincent A. Marinkovich, M.D.
Diplomate, American Board of Allergy and Clinical Immunology
Clinical Associate Professor, Stanford Medical School

PREFACE

WHAT THIS BOOK CAN DO FOR YOU

The field of allergy was just beginning to expand in 1983, when Dr. Alan Levin and I coauthored *The Type 1/Type 2 Allergy Relief Program*, which described two types of allergies: traditional and environmental.

Many changes have occurred in the last decade. One is that environmental allergy is now known as MCS, or multiple chemical sensitivity. Even though MCS is not, by strict definition, an allergy, it behaves like one in many ways, and the environmental specialists who treat it are generally allergists. This book will focus mainly on classic allergy but will also bring you up to date on MCS.

Part I explains what allergy is and which symptoms may— or may not—be caused by allergies. Part II describes the newest tests and treatments, the most effective medications, and how to cope with their side effects. You'll also learn what kind of physician offers the best treatment for you and how to find such a person.

Controlling allergenic substances in the home, protecting your skin, and dealing with food allergies are the subjects of Part III. Parts IV and V cover asthma and MCS, and Part VI discusses alternative therapies and ways to reduce stress.

The last decade has seen great improvements in diagnostic techniques, medication, and available knowledge, but allergy is still a controversial illness, affecting greater numbers of people than ever before.

More than 50 million Americans—one in five—have some

sort of allergic illness, and unlike many other medical problems, allergy has no specific therapy (except avoidance) that works for everyone. Trial-and-error is still the best way to determine what products and procedures will help you.

This book is meant to supplement the advice of your doctor, not to replace it. The use of medication, treatment, or other measures should be undertaken only on advice of your physician, and for this reason, the author and publisher disclaim any responsibility for whatever consequences result from reading this book. Only a physician can offer medical tests and treatment, and with proper guidance, only you can take steps to reduce stress in your life, improve your general health, and do everything possible to avoid the offending substances.

"Learn to live with your allergies," a doctor once told me, but that's not the whole story. You can conquer them, too. Let this sourcebook be your compendium of the most practical information known about the subject, including the latest discoveries, theories, and medical breakthroughs.

PART I

KNOWLEDGE CAN HEAL

My dad used to say I was allergic to cleaning my room. Little did he know how right he was—stirring up dust mites and mold spores was the last thing my sensitive sinuses needed.

Fortunately, I've since learned ways to vacuum my rugs without sneezing, weed the garden without wheezing, and gobble shrimps without blossoming into a rash. That's what allergies are: abnormal reactions to everyday substances such as dust, pollen, common foods, or chemicals.

And the more you know about the subject, the quicker you can take charge of your health.

CHAPTER 1

WHAT IS ALLERGY?

Medically speaking, an allergic response occurs when the immune system, poised to rout bacteria and viruses, goes haywire and reacts to harmless substances such as cat dander or dust. These substances are called allergens.

The body then produces protein molecules called antibodies to fight the allergens. The antibodies attach themselves to mast cells, tiny time bombs plentiful in the respiratory and gastrointestinal tracts. When the mast cells explode, they release a load of chemicals, including histamine, a powerful substance that causes symptoms.

Allergic rhinitis or hay fever, the most common form of allergy, involves the respiratory system—nasal cavity, mouth, throat, bronchi, lungs, and diaphragm—and often brings on its own mini-version of Niagara Falls.

But there are other types of allergy that affect various parts of the body. The area where symptoms appear is called a shock organ or target organ and may differ in each individual. For instance, milk may cause a skin rash in one person, abdominal cramps in another, asthma in a third.

The eyes, ears, and gastrointestinal tract are other common shock organs and, less commonly, the heart, bladder, blood vessels, kidney, muscles, joints, brain, and central nervous system. A person's shock organs can change with age. A baby girl's eczema, for example, might develop into hay fever as she grows.

WHY ME?

Children often wonder why their friends can cuddle kittens without getting hives, or play in the grass without getting a runny nose, and ask themselves: "Why me? Why am I different?"

The answer is a bit complicated. Many factors play a role in the development of allergy, but the strongest is heredity. When one parent is allergic, the child runs a 50 percent chance of inheriting the tendency. When both parents are allergic, the odds jump to 75 percent, although the child may not inherit the same symptoms or sensitivities to the same substances. Even if neither parent is allergic, anyone can become allergic at any time, if three conditions prevail.

1. The tendency to produce large quantities of Immunoglobulin E or IgE, a specific antibody present in allergic reactions.

2. Repeated exposure to the allergen, the substance that causes a reaction. Almost anything inhaled, eaten, touched, or injected into the body can become an allergen.

3. Sufficient potency and duration of exposure.

When all three factors are in play, the process is called sensitization. Say, for instance, that you're stung by a bee for the first time. You have no response, except maybe an "ouch!" But because you inherited the tendency to produce IgE, these antibodies form in your blood and circulate throughout your body. In other words, you've become sensitized.

Sometime later you get a second sting. Your immune system considers the bee venom a foreign invader and mobilizes the IgE antibodies to fight it, thus starting the chemical process that causes symptoms. Sensitization can happen after a single exposure or after many years of exposure, depending on how long a person's body takes to produce antibodies.

A few unfortunate souls acquire acute, potentially lethal sensitivity, especially to insect stings, certain foods such as peanuts or shellfish, sulfites and other additives, and drugs such as penicillin and aspirin.

For these people, the result of even a single bee sting or a peanut is anaphylaxis, a frightening condition that intensifies rapidly. It starts with breathing difficulty and a drop in blood pressure, and proceeds to unconsciousness, coma, and even death. Fortunately, anaphylaxis is rare and can be controlled and prevented. (See Chapter 6.)

OVER THE THRESHOLD

In most cases, even after you become sensitized, not every encounter with an allergen will bring on a reaction. If you're allergic to strawberries, for instance, the question is: How many strawberries will trigger symptoms? One or two may not do it, but that third piece of fruit, because you've been "primed," will push you right over your allergy threshold. Doctors call this the priming effect.

Think of it as the proverbial straw that breaks the camel's back. You can endure a certain amount of exposure to pollen, molds, or other allergens without having symptoms. But once your system gets primed—that is, loaded to the point where you exceed your threshold—you begin to react.

Take a second example. You may be allergic to house dust, but have no reaction when the concentration of dust in the air is low. Change the bedding and you start to sniffle.

A combination of allergens can also shoot you over the threshold. Say you're watching television in a room with musty wallpaper. Mold spores are in the air, but not bothering you. Suddenly, your cat comes in, jumps on your lap, and sets you off on a sneezing fit. Separately, the molds and cat dander might not affect you, but together—whammo!

Another factor is air pollution. You may or may not be allergic to the chemicals themselves, but their effect is the same: to prime the body, that is, to make the mucous membranes more permeable and raise IgE levels. The result is that when even a small amount of allergen strikes, your immune system is so receptive, it bursts into action.

Particular pollutants to watch out for are: natural gas (methane); PCBs (polychlorinated biphenyls) found in insulators, paints, and varnishes; smog (ozone); car exhaust (carbon monoxide); and tobacco smoke. A recent Swedish survey showed that mothers who smoked while pregnant quadrupled their chances of having an allergic baby.

Incidentally, there's some evidence that keeping a child solely on breast milk for six months may increase the child's resistance to food allergies later. Breast-feeding also protects the infant by delaying exposure to foods such as cow's milk, which often causes allergies.

Solid foods should be introduced gradually into the baby's diet so that any allergy will be easily found. The most common reactions are to cow's milk, wheat, eggs, chocolate, corn, and citrus fruits. Rice cereal is a safe introduction to solid foods.

THE FIRST STEP

Before you rush off to an allergist, check with your primary-care doctor. Get a thorough physical exam, and remember that "allergy" can be a handy crutch for physicians who can't find anything wrong with you. Be sure to ask questions (see Chapter 4) before accepting a diagnosis of allergy.

Technically, every human being has the potential to become allergic. People with no allergies have never exceeded their allergy thresholds. That's one reason why allergy shots work. They don't eliminate the allergy; rather, they raise your threshold so you can tolerate more of the substance before you get symptoms.

This threshold can vary during your lifetime. Emotional stress, a viral illness, fatigue, exposure to chemical irritants, overexertion, and severe weather conditions can lower your threshold and make you more reactive.

Eliminating tension, improving diet, and enjoying general good health can sometimes raise the threshold. Even age can help. One of the lesser known advantages of the golden years is that the immune system's efficiency begins to wane, and those IgE antibodies are less and less eager to challenge invading allergens. That's why older people have fewer allergic problems.

By now you've begun to realize that allergy is a complex subject, an unwanted side effect of a civilization that brings us a constant influx of chemicals, products, and technologies. Those same technologies, however, enable doctors and scientists to explore new theories, conduct more effective studies, improve medication, and, in general, offer better treatment and broader horizons of hope to all who need it.

CHAPTER 2

ALLERGIC RHINITIS/ HAY FEVER

Jennifer B. locked the front door, climbed into her Chevy, and drove to the church where she was meeting friends to work on a rummage sale.

Shortly after she began sorting through boxes of old clothing, her nose started to run—and run—and kept on running, until finally she had to leave.

That evening, she told her husband, "I had a hay fever attack in the vestry today. I think I'm allergic to church."

Approximately 40 million Americans—one in six persons—have some form of allergic rhinitis, better known as hay fever. Technically, rhinitis means inflammation of the nasal mucous membrane, or, in simpler terms, a runny nose.

The most common cause is inhaling airborne substances derived from natural sources: house dust, pollens, mold spores, animal and insect emanations. Along with drippy noses, airborne allergens may bring on itchy eyes, sore throats, ear infections, headaches, stomach cramps, skin rashes, hives, fatigue, irritability, urinary frequency, diarrhea, and asthma. Symptoms can appear at all stages of life, but 70 percent of patients develop hay fever before they reach age 30.

THREE TYPES

Allergic rhinitis falls into three categories:

Seasonal

These include reactions to tree pollens in early spring, grasses in late spring to midsummer, and weeds in late summer and early fall. Despite what you've heard, bright-colored flowers rarely cause symptoms because their pollens are spread by insects rather than the wind. Equally misleading is the term "hayfever." It may occasionally refer to hay, a dried grass, but has nothing to do with fever.

Not all seasonal reactions are caused by pollen. Fertilizer, for instance, is applied mainly in spring and fall and contains large amounts of animal dander (old skin scales). Damp leaves in late fall tend to grow molds. Children returning to school in September may confront dusty desks and classrooms.

Perennial (year round)

Common triggers are molds, house dust mites, cockroach particles, cat and dog dander, certain foods, and chemicals. Jennifer may have been reacting to molds and dust stirred into the air from the old clothes, or to dust or molds in the church itself.

Episodic

Some allergens occur randomly and unpredictably, such as insect stings and poison ivy.

NONALLERGIC RHINITIS

Persistent nasal congestion and discharge are sometimes mistakenly diagnosed as allergic rhinitis. They may, however, be due to sinusitis or other respiratory infection, bronchitis, nasal polyps, swollen adenoids, or a mechanical obstruction such as a deviated septum.

Nonallergic rhinitis can also be traced to "rebound congestion" from use of nasal sprays more than twice daily for three consecutive days. Hormones and oral contraceptives, certain medications (beta-blockers such as Lopressor and Inderal, vasodilators, and reserpine derivatives), or drugs, particularly cocaine, can cause runny noses. Still other sources include sudden temperature changes, alcoholic beverages (mainly beer and wine), air pollution, eating spicy foods, emotional upsets, and fatigue.

Strong scents such as perfumes, aerosol sprays, household cleaners, laundry detergent, and cigarette smoke can trigger symptoms that may be allergies, but are more likely to be reactions to irritants rather than allergens, because they don't involve the immune system.

Short-term use of saltwater nose drops or sprays can sometimes relieve symptoms of nonallergic rhinitis. If your nose is running badly, an antihistamine with a decongestant may help. (See Chapter 6.)

The common cold is a familiar form of nonallergic rhinitis. Symptoms are a low-grade fever, a thick yellowish nasal discharge, and a general malaise that lasts three to seven days. Unlike allergy, which is not contagious, cold germs can easily spread to other members of the family.

TREATMENT

A hay fever episode is characterized by sudden sneezing, a watery nasal discharge, puffy eyes, and a sense of fatigue that can last for weeks. The most telling clue to allergy is a cause-and-effect relationship. Are your symptoms a result of exposure to a suspected allergen?

If your discomfort is severe, seek medical help, preferably from your primary-care doctor, who may or may not recommend an allergist. Symptoms of allergy often mimic symptoms of other diseases, including some serious ones. These diseases must be ruled out before allergy is ruled in.

The doctor should first review your complete history, asking how and when your symptoms occur, how long you've had them, home and work conditions, and so on. A thorough physical checkup should include a nasal smear (you blow your nose onto a plastic sheet and the specimen is transferred to a slide). A microscopic exam of secretions may show high numbers of eosinophils, special white blood cells present in allergy. The physician should also examine the mucous membranes of your nose. They usually appear swollen, pale, and bluish in allergic persons.

If your doctor sends you to an allergist for skin-testing, diluted extracts of allergens will be injected under the skin or applied to scratches on your back or upper arm. Positive results— raised welts surrounded by redness—show a high level of IgE antibodies, the standard indication of allergy.

Blood tests such as the RAST (radioallergosorbent test) are also used to determine IgE levels. (See Chapter 5.)

COMMON TRIGGERS

Airborne inhalants top the list of triggers of allergic rhinitis. Medical treatment is always advisable, but simpler, less expensive measures can help as well. These (and the chemicals covered in Chapter 17) are the main troublemakers:

House Dust

The major allergens in house dust are mite feces, affectionately known in allergy circles as "mite poo," and pieces of dead mites. These particles are so tiny that they float into the air whenever you fluff a pillow, pat a stuffed animal, or walk across a carpet.

Dust mites live and multiply in warm, humid places. They eat specks of skin and dander and thrive in rugs, mattresses, upholstered furniture, clothing, closets, drawers, and car seats.

House dust may also contain human skin flakes, fabric fibers, cat and dog dander, mold spores, food particles, cockroach body parts and feces, and other debris. The number of dust mite sufferers is steadily and rapidly growing.

WHAT YOU CAN DO. Take a tour of your own house. Ask yourself such questions as: How clean is the air? Do I have a lot of decorative doodads and dustcatchers? What objects can I eliminate? If I run my finger over most surfaces, do I get dust?

Then give top priority to cleaning up your indoor environment as soon as possible. (See Chapter 8.)

Pollen

Trees, grasses, and weeds are the prime sources of pollen, a fine powderlike material that contains the male gametes or plant sperm, the fertilizing element of plants. In order for certain plants to reproduce, pollen must be discharged into the air and transmitted. Pollens from trees and weeds can travel many miles, even to the heart of a major urbanized city.

Ragweed and grasses are the most common and potent sources. A single ragweed plant can release a million pollen grains a day, particles so light they can be carried by the wind as far as 400 miles. Ragweed grows almost everywhere in the United States except along parts of the West Coast, the southernmost tip of Florida, and the northern tip of Maine.

WHAT YOU CAN DO. Most allergists don't recommend moving away. Any area with green foliage has pollen, and chances are that you'll develop new allergies in your new location. Your best tactic is to stay at home during the peak of the pollen season with closed windows and air conditioning that recirculates indoor air only.

If you're making plans for the day, check the weather forecast, not the pollen count. By the time air samples have been collected, counted, and reported, they're at least 24 hours old.

Your best bet is to bypass dry, sunny, and windy days and look for fog, drizzle, and rain, which help clear the air—although mold spores may be higher right after a rain.

As a general rule, don't venture outside between 5 A.M. and 10 A.M., when most pollination is in full bloom. Ragweed pollen counts, however, reach their peak between 11 A.M. and 12 noon.

Breathe through your nose—it's a natural air filter. Avoid bright sunlight as it puts extra strain on already irritated and watering eyes. Dark glasses can help, and you can remove pollens by rinsing your eyes with artificial tears.

Pollen counts drop substantially by late afternoon, so that's the best time for walking and outdoor sports. Do your gardening in the evening, or assign yard work to someone else. Keep your lawn clipped, no higher than 1½ inches. A lawn that grows freely will go to seed and release pollen. Water the soil regularly to keep down molds and dust.

If you must mow grass or rake leaves, wear a filter mask. An inexpensive one from the pharmacy or hardware store will do. Throw it away after each use, or pollens will collect on the outside and cause problems when you try to reuse it.

Don't bring ragweed-related flowers such as daisies, dahlias, and chrysanthemums into the house, and be wary of certain foods. Some ragweed-sensitive souls develop mouth and throat swelling after eating melons, zucchini, cucumber, sunflower seeds, or sipping chamomile tea.

In early spring, the trees to avoid are elm, maple, birch, olive, sycamore, western red cedar, poplar, ash, oak, walnut, beech, cypress, and hickory. In late spring and early summer, stay away from such pollinating grasses as timothy, redtop, orchard, and Bermuda. From late summer to fall, be wary of these weeds: sagebrush, tumbleweed, Russian thistle, sorrel, plantain, pigweed, box elder, and the ubiquitous ragweed.

Choose "sneezeless" plants for your garden. Pine, plum, magnolia, and dogwood trees and colorful flowers such as azaleas, tulips, and peonies are excellent choices.

If you're ever exposed to a blast of pollen, shower and rinse your clothes as soon as possible. Don't dry them on outdoor lines where they can attract more pollen. Wash your hair before bedtime, as pollen clings to it and can rub off on sheets and pillows and trigger allergies overnight.

Reduce—or better yet, stop altogether—consumption of alcohol during allergy season. It stimulates mucus production and dilates blood vessels, worsening runny nose and congestion. Tobacco smoke, of course, is another potent irritant.

Try to vacation at the beach, where vegetation is scarce and coastal breezes blow pollen inland. Hot, dry areas such as rural Arizona have low pollen counts. If your time and money permit, take an ocean cruise to Europe. The sea air is fresh and invigorating, and the continent has little or no ragweed.

Molds

Molds (fungi or mildew) are tiny parasites that live on decaying plant or animal matter. They grow almost everywhere—on soil, wood, fabrics, and foods. Some are cultured commercially for the production of drugs such as penicillin. Some are edible, such as yeast and mushrooms, and many are used to produce certain foods: cheese, soy sauce, yogurt, wine, and beer, for example.

Molds thrive in warm, moist darkness. Dryness is their enemy. They reproduce by forming spores (asexual reproductive cells) and sending them into the air all year round, but mainly in the warmer months. The spores do best in wet climates and, like pollen, can be carried great distances by the wind.

WHAT YOU CAN DO. Remove leaves, grass clippings, and compost from the area surrounding your house. Avoid damp cellars and barns, wooded cabins and resorts, lumber mills, granaries, antique and thrift shops, and bargain sales in musty basements and garages. Store fireplace wood outside the house.

If you must go camping in the woods, wash your sleeping bag in very hot water before leaving home. Search for a relatively clear spot away from rotted logs and vegetation.

Don't play or work with soil or sand, and stay indoors on

wet or windy days. Keep your home dry. Repair moisture leaks in your roof, walls, and plumbing, and be wary of dry rot. Seal off crawl spaces or use black plastic to prevent the spread of mold in them.

Say good-bye to foolish sentiment. Clear out old clothing stored in the attic and discard mildewed scrapbooks, photos, and love letters.

Mold can grow on bathroom walls, behind peeling wallpaper, and on stalks and leaves of indoor plants. You'll find it in room vaporizers, humidifiers, rugs, mattresses, feather and foam rubber pillows, stuffed furniture, and air conditioners.

There is often a brief burst of mold spores when the air conditioner starts running, so you may want to turn it on, leave the room for 15 minutes to give the molds time to disperse, then return. The same with your car. Close the vents and run the air conditioner with the car windows open for a few minutes before you get in.

Animal Dander

Animal dander is the skin, saliva, dandruff, and urine from an animal, not the animal's hair. The commonly held belief that short-haired dogs are less allergenic than long-haired dogs is a myth. So is the legend that poodles don't cause allergies, although they may have less dander because they're washed and groomed more frequently than other breeds.

Sixty percent of American households have pets, and one in four persons scratch-tested for allergy will react positively to dog and cat dander, especially the latter. Light, airy cat dander tends to linger long after the animal has left the scene. Dogs are somewhat less potent. Also, some people may be sensitized to a single type of dog but able to tolerate other breeds.

Puppies and kittens have no old skin to shed and therefore less dander. This may explain why some children can tolerate baby animals but not mature ones. Cats and dogs often roam through grassy areas where pollen clings to their fur, leading some people to assume they're allergic to pets when they're actually reacting to the pollens—or in some cases, to tiny insects that live on their pets.

Horses and farm animals provide strong allergens, and our feathered friends aren't always friendly, although it's the dander on their feathers that causes problems. Animal allergies carry over to all related products: fur coats, horsehair upholstery, down comforters, wool and mohair sweaters.

WHAT YOU CAN DO. Ventilate your house. Desirable as energy efficiency is, an insulated home retains 40 times more pet allergen than a noninsulated home. Air filters help slightly, but pet emanations are remarkably durable and can stay in furniture, carpets, draperies, and heating ducts for as long as six months.

A better solution is to make your bedroom off limits to pets. Better still, keep pets out of the house altogether and always groom them outdoors. Bathe them with mild shampoo at least once a week to reduce dander, and be sure to wash your hands after touching or petting them.

If you or your children are sensitive to cats, dogs, birds, or other furry or feathered creatures, consider replacing the pets with tropical fish, turtles, lizards, and yes, even snakes.

CHAPTER 3

PLAYING DETECTIVE— CHECKLIST OF SYMPTOMS

Vicki M. could hardly wait for Saturday night. She'd been dating Doug, the class president, for several weeks, and now at last he was taking her to the prom. Everything went well until they reached the dance floor. A few minutes into the fox trot, Vicki was mortified to find that the right side of her face was breaking out in large red welts.

After much speculation, Doug remembered that his dog had been licking his cheek just before he left home, and that Vicki was allergic to dogs—and dog saliva. They both washed their faces with soap and water, danced a little less romantically, and Vicki's hives subsided. An evening that could have been a disaster was saved by sharp sleuthing.

Playing detective can help solve your problems as well. The two most important factors in allergy relief are (1) diagnosis and (2) avoidance. Obviously, you need an accurate diagnosis—that is, you need to know what's causing your symptoms—in order to know what to avoid.

Before seeing your primary-care doctor, arm yourself with as many facts and observations as possible. Be sure to bring a list of all medications you're taking. Beta-agonists, such as

Proventil, thyroid hormones (Cytomel, Thyrolar), and oral contraceptives can have side effects that imitate allergy.

Do you have any of the following symptoms? Mark the ones that apply:

RESPIRATORY

NOSE

Sneezing, with runny or congested nose

Watery nasal discharge

Postnasal drip

Loss of sense of smell

Sinus headache

Nasal crease (a line across lower part of nose due to excess upward rubbing, sometimes called the "allergic salute")

Nasal polyps (watery swellings in the nose that can obstruct breathing)

Frequent nosebleeds

THROAT

Sore throat

Loss of voice

Croup (coughing and difficulty breathing, especially in infants and children)

CHEST

Chronic cough

Wheezing or shortness of breath

EYES

Itching, watery, or puffy eyes

Conjunctivitis or pinkeye (red, swollen eyes; crusty lids)

Shiners (dark circles due to swollen blood vessels under eyes)

Sensitivity to light

EARS

Pain or pressure in ears
Ear infection
Sensitivity to loud sounds
Decreased hearing due to fluid in the middle ear

GASTROINTESTINAL

MOUTH

Canker sores
Swollen, chapped lips
Bad breath
Geographical tongue (a patchy tongue, resembling a map)
Loss of taste
Itchy palate

STOMACH

Abdominal pain, cramps
Bloating, belching, heartburn
Diarrhea/constipation
Nausea, vomiting

GENITOURINARY

Incontinence
Painful or frequent urination
Vaginal itching

SKIN

Eczema (a dry, itchy rash)
Hives, local or generalized

SYSTEMIC (Happening in the Whole Body)

Chills
Rapid heartbeat
Light-headedness
Tiredness, fatigue
General malaise
Irritability
Depression

Here are some questions you should be prepared to answer:

• What other symptoms do you have?

• Are you oversensitive to heat, cold, or temperature changes?

• Are symptoms worse in mornings and better in evenings? (This might suggest allergy to bedding, pets, or house dust whereas the opposite pattern might be linked to substances at work.)

• Are symptoms worse at certain times of the year? (This could indicate seasonal allergy, for example, to pollens in spring and summer, to molds in the fall, to gas heating fumes in winter.)

• Do symptoms appear at a particular time or location?

• Do they change when you go indoors or outdoors?

• How long do they last?

• Do you notice an absence of symptoms in the mountains? At the beach? In any other places?

• Do you feel better when you skip a meal? (This may suggest a food allergy.)

• Have you noticed reactions to particular foods? (Describe reactions. What foods?)

- Do you feel tired much of the time?
- Are your symptoms worse when you're exposed to house dust? Molds? Animal dander?
- Do you have blood relatives with allergy?

Your primary-care doctor needs to know everything you can think of about yourself and your symptoms, and will ask a lot of general questions. The allergist, if you see one, will quiz you even more thoroughly, delving into your diet, cosmetics, clothing, furnishings and appliances, medication, exercise habits, house-cleaning routine, occupation and hobbies, family relationships, family health problems, and possible stress factors. The more precise your information, the better. You may want to bring along your spouse or lover, or in a child's case, a sibling, who may be able to add insights and observations.

Try to be patient with the doctor's probing and grilling, no matter how personal. Every question has its reasons, and the answers contain the clues that will lead to solving your illness. (If the doctor or an assistant does not ask a barrage of questions, change doctors.)

Playing detective can be challenging and frustrating, but the rewards make it worthwhile. Sherlock Holmes said it well: "The game is afoot."

GATHERING CLUES

If you like mysteries, why not tackle your own case? An allergy may be as obvious as a runny nose every spring, or a rash whenever you eat seafood. But if the source of your problem is elusive, try keeping a record of your symptoms for several weeks. You may find a pattern that points to one or more substances.

Here's how to do it. Make a simple chart like this:

---

1. TIME/DATE/LOCATION

   _____

2. OBSERVATIONS (what you touched, ate, smelled prior to having symptoms)

   _____

3. SYMPTOMS

   _____

4. POSSIBLE ALLERGENS (including pills, nose drops or sprays, any medication you're taking)

   _____

Repeat the chart for as many pages as necessary. Set aside a special time to fill it out, probably just before bedtime. Be accurate and consistent, and don't skip a day. Keep in mind that the *absence* of symptoms in a particular locale may also provide clues.

Your own observations combined with the doctor's wisdom and experience should give a fairly good indication of what's bothering you. Depending on the severity of your symptoms, however, you may still want to be tested. (See Chapter 5.)

LATE-PHASE REACTIONS

Would-be Sherlocks take note: Not all allergic reactions are immediate. While most occur within minutes of exposure, others may be delayed 3–12 hours or more, due to a later release of chemicals from the mast cells.

Some late-phase reactions are familiar. Many of us know from firsthand knowledge that poison oak and ivy can generate a rash 12–48 hours after contact. Migraine headaches can come on 3–6 hours after eating certain foods, and venom from an insect sting or spider bite can, in rare cases, take up to a week to cause symptoms.

Medications or reactions to immunizations such as for rubella (German measles) can also be latecomers. Delayed symptoms can range from a rash or hives to respiratory obstruction and/or severe systemic problems: fever, swelling, hemorrhaging, joint pains, or swollen lymph glands.

Late-phase reactions obviously present a greater challenge to the cause-and-effect seeker, but when all clues lead to a question mark, it's time to call in the experts.

PART II

WHAT ALLERGISTS DO

Let's assume that you've seen your primary-care doctor, learned you have allergies, and are thinking about consulting a specialist. Naturally, you wonder: Will the results justify the time and expense?

Consider this. An allergist:

- Can offer the kind of consultation and testing that will help pinpoint the cause of your symptoms and determine the degree of sensitivity.
- Can provide nonsedating antihistamines, cortisone nasal sprays, and other prescription medication and alert you to possible side effects.
- Can provide expert advice on cleaning up your environment, and suggest specific products that will help "clear the air."
- Can treat you with immunotherapy in the form of injections.
- Can prescribe an ANA-kit or EpiPen (injectable epinephrine) that could save your life in case of an anaphylactic reaction.
- Can offer diets—mold-free, wheat-free, or whatever—as well as nutritional information custom-tailored to your needs.

That is what allergists do that other doctors, for the most part, don't do. There's no question that you'll have to devote time and energy to getting a diagnosis and following through with treatment, even if it's as simple as taking avoidance measures.

Medical costs can run high, but most health insurance will cover traditional methods. More experimental tests and treatments may not be covered, so you and your doctor should discuss this in advance. You don't need surprises later.

CHAPTER 4

DOCTOR SHOPPING— DO'S AND DON'TS

Allergy, unfortunately, attracts its share of eccentrics and unorthodox doctors, and while many are well-meaning and effective, others are more mercenary than merciful and may do you serious harm. That's why it's important to be a savvy consumer. Choose an allergist as carefully as you'd hire a live-in housekeeper or a babysitter.

Here's how to start. Do:

• Ask your primary-care doctor for a recommendation.

• Get names from other doctors, dentists, friends, pharmacists—anyone you trust and respect.

• Collect at least three to six names. The more people you talk to, the bigger your field of choice. When several names float to the top, skim off the cream.

• Take your time. Find out all you can about each doctor. (See next section for questions to ask.)

• Check credentials. Call the American Board of Medical Specialties, 800-776-CERT weekdays, 9 A.M. to 6 P.M. EST, to find out if a doctor is board-certified. "Yes" doesn't necessarily mean more competence, but it does mean that the physician has taken an additional three to seven years of training and has passed a rigorous exam.

- Look for the person's name in *Questionable Doctors*, a book listing all doctors disciplined by their state medical boards since 1991. The book is available at most libraries, or you can get the names of doctors disciplined in your state by sending $15 to Public Citizen, Publications Dept. PLO394, 2000 P Street NW, Suite 600, Washington, DC 20036. For more information, call 202-833-3000.

- Educate yourself about allergy. Know which tests and treatments are considered safe and effective and which are controversial.

At the same time, observe the following don'ts:

- Don't wait until you're too ill to make a careful, unhurried choice.

- Don't call the county medical society or a doctor-referral service. The names they supply may not have been approved or evaluated by an objective board. Some doctors even pay to be listed with a referral service.

- Don't let your fingers walk through the Yellow Pages. The decision is too important to pick a name because it catches your eye, or because the doctor's office is nearby.

- Don't necessarily take the first name you hear. Even your primary-care doctor may not be altogether objective about his medical school classmate or his wife's second cousin.

WHAT TO ASK

Getting at least three referrals from other doctors, friends, and acquaintances shouldn't be difficult. People who have been helped by a doctor are usually happy to pass along a recommendation.

When seeking information, do so in person whenever possible. Face-to-face conversations tend to be more honest and thoughtful than hasty phone chats.

Here are 10 questions you may want to ask:

1. If a member of your family had allergies, whom would you recommend and why?

2. Is Dr. X a traditional allergist, an environmental specialist, or a combination?

3. Does Dr. X seem to keep up with new developments?

4. Does Dr. X answer questions thoroughly, cheerfully, and in language you understand?

5. Does Dr. X explain the tests and treatment options?

6. Does Dr. X treat more than half his patients with immunotherapy? (If so, consider another doctor. Immunotherapy is warranted in less than 50 percent of allergy patients.)

7. Is Dr. X easy to talk to?

8. Do you have to wait long in the office?

9. Will Dr. X answer questions on the phone?

10. Are Dr. X's fees reasonable?

At this point, it would be nice if you could meet and talk to doctors the way you would a prospective contractor or housekeeper, but most are too busy to be "interviewed." You can, however, make an appointment for a new-patient consultation/evaluation that will cost from $50 to $200. Be sure to ask the fee when you make your initial phone call. You might also ask about testing technique, usually a good indication of how conservative a doctor is—or isn't. As an experiment, I called five allergists from the Yellow Pages and asked their office assistants: What kind of testing does the doctor do, skin tests or RAST?

These were the answers:

"Dr. A only does skin tests because the American Academy of Allergy and Immunology says skin tests are more sensitive than RAST."

"Dr. B does three panels of skin-testing on the back, including one for foods. No RAST."

"Dr. C does both, but prefers RAST. It's more precise and reliable than skin tests."

"Dr. D doesn't do either skin tests or RAST. We only do intradermal testing—injections under the skin so we can get a whole body reaction."

"Dr. E does all kinds of testing, including intradermal and provocative-neutralization. He evaluates each patient to see which he'll use."

Confused? Don't despair. If you have simple hay fever, any one of the five doctors could help, although I'd question Dr. B, who uses skin tests to determine food allergies. They're not reliable for foods, except to give possible clues or when there's an immediate, life-threatening reaction. I'd also find out more about Dr. D, who doesn't use either skin tests or RAST.

If your symptoms are more complicated and include chemical sensitivities (see Chapter 15), you'd probably do better with Doctors C, D, or E. The important thing is to learn all you can about the various tests so you can make an informed decision.

Before hanging up on that first call, ask if the doctor is willing to bill your insurance company or, if applicable, will take Medicare or Medicaid assignment. You may also want to find out about office hours, location, public transportation, and parking facilities.

THE CONSULTATION

You're about to meet the doctor, and there's no reason to be apprehensive. Don't forget: *You're* the one seeking advice and treatment, and you're paying well for those services. It's up to the doctor to convey to you that he or she can deliver what you need, and it's up to you to impress the doctor with three facts: You're informed, you're prepared, and you're willing to play an active role in getting well.

As soon as you enter the doctor's office, make a few mental notes. How long do you have to wait? Are the staff friendly and courteous? Is there a "No Smoking" sign in the waiting room?

(This shows the doctor's commitment to the comfort of all patients.) Does the doctor seem cordial and concerned or rushed
and reserved?

Answer all the doctor's questions about your medical history, and share the results of your sleuthing, but don't agree to
be tested, medicated, or treated until you've had a complete
physical exam from either your primary-care doctor or the allergist.

Your next step is to ask:

- How do you plan to test me?

- For what substances? (Be sure everything you suspect is included.)

- Why did you choose that (those) particular method(s)?

- What will you learn from the tests?

- What will be the treatment options?

- Could you explain your fee schedule?

If the answers are clear, logical, and satisfying, make an appointment to be tested. If the answers leave you confused or the
doctor seems resentful, feel free to try the second name on your
list. Be patient with whomever you finally choose. Immunotherapy can take months to show results.

Some allergists can make you feel like a jelly jar on an as-
sembly line. They see you once, then turn you over to their
testers, technicians, and nurses, who perform their separate
functions, provide you with sheets of written instructions, and
send you out into the world. If this arrangement doesn't work
for you, ask to see the doctor and explain your dissatisfaction.
Remember: You always have the option to change physicians.

CHAPTER 5

TESTING, TESTING

The important fact to remember about allergy tests is that they are only useful when correlated with your symptoms and your medical history. *Test results must never be the sole bases for allergy diagnosis and/or treatment.*

At best, tests confirm what the doctor has already surmised, but they can be misleading. A perfectly healthy person may show positive reactions to test allergens yet have no symptoms. Conversely, a person who tests negative to house dust may have a sneezing fit at the first buzz of a vacuum cleaner. This could be due to any number of variables, from lab errors to biological differences.

Tests to determine IgE antibodies—usual indicators of allergy—are either in vivo, in or on the living body, or in vitro, in a test tube or artificial environment. Skin tests are in vivo; RAST tests are in vitro, performed in the lab using a blood sample.

SKIN TESTS

Skin tests are the most popular diagnostic tool, and according to the *Journal of the American Medical Association* (*JAMA*), they're "the least time-consuming and expensive" and the "most revealing tests for disclosing specific sensitivities."

The American Academy of Allergy and Immunology (AAA&I), the nation's largest professional medical society representing allergists, immunologists, and related professionals, agrees: [Skin tests] are quicker than RAST, less expensive, and better standardized."

Research is ongoing at the Food and Drug Administration (FDA), but because of limited funds and higher priorities, only a few extracts of dust and pollen have been standardized for use in tests and treatment (see Chapter 7). The advantages of standardization are that you can count on safe, high-quality products, and you can change doctors without having to change injection dosage.

There's no way to prepare for skin tests, but you'll be asked to stop certain medications, especially antihistamines, for two to seven days beforehand.

Three types of skin test are available. Some doctors use only one method; others combine them:

Scratch or Prick Test

A technician places dilute drops of suspected allergens on the skin of the upper arm or back, then scratches them lightly with a sterile needle. (Some technicians use a boardlike device that they press to the skin to apply eight extracts at once.)

After 10 to 30 minutes (allergists use different dilutions that have slightly varying time intervals,) a reddish wheal, like a mosquito bite, may appear. Its size indicates the degree of sensitivity to the allergen. Reactions can also occur several hours later, or even the next day.

Intradermal Test

Minute amounts of allergen are injected just below the surface of the skin. You feel only a tiny sting. Again, you'll wait 10 to 30 minutes for the response to be measured.

Intradermal tests are more sensitive than scratch tests and

are sometimes used to confirm scratch test results, especially for stinging insects and drugs.

Patch Test

Small absorbent pads containing allergen are affixed to the skin with nonallergenic tape, left there for 24–72 hours, then evaluated. You'll be asked not to bathe that area or to engage in vigorous physical activity. If you have severe pain or itching, remove the patch immediately and call your doctor.

Patch tests are particularly helpful in diagnosing allergic contact dermatitis (ACD), a rash that comes from direct skin contact. Some critics say skin tests are too sensitive and give positive readings where no allergy exists. Also, the readings are not reliable for infants and people over 60. Nevertheless, skin tests have proven to be relatively accurate for most substances except foods and are generally safe. The major risk with any in vivo allergy test is an anaphylactic reaction, but it's rare.

The cost of skin-testing can range from $200 to $700, which includes $3 to $4 per allergen. Almost all medical insurance covers it.

BLOOD TESTS

Insurers haven't always been willing to pay for the RAST (radioallergosorbent test), which may or may not cost more than skin-testing, depending on the number of substances tested and the doctor's markup of lab charges. This once-controversial diagnostic tool has graduated to general acceptance, however, with FDA approval and even a cautious nod from the conservative *JAMA*.

Like skin tests, RASTs have benefits and limitations. According to Dr. Edward O'Connell, professor of pediatrics, allergy/immunology at the Mayo School of Medicine, "RAST is practical, easy on the patient, and effective even if a patient has a body rash or other symptoms, or is taking antihistamines. Some of the newer medications, especially Hismanal, can affect skin-test results for up to two months."

Experts agree that while skin tests sometimes give false positives, especially to foods, RAST can give false negatives—that is, it may miss substances you are allergic to.

RAST has many spin-offs, such as ELISA (enzyme-linked immuno-assay test), known for its ability to detect the human immunodeficiency virus (HIV); and PRIST (paper radioimmunosorbent test), which measures the total number of IgE antibodies in the blood.

Dr. Vincent A. Marinkovich, diplomate, American Board of Allergy and Clinical Immunology, has helped develop a version of RAST called MAST—Multiple Antigen Simultaneous Testing.

"MAST is more comprehensive and sensitive than RAST," he explains. "RAST deals with single allergens and MAST can test 38 at a time. It's not diagnostic for foods, but it can direct you to areas where there may be problems." (See Chapter 10 for food testing.)

Having been skin-tested all my life, and being quite familiar with my allergies, I decided to try MAST and check its accuracy. Dr. Marinkovich agreed to take a blood sample, and knowing nothing about me or my medical history, he ran it through the lab.

The results were impressive; I'd say 8.5 on a scale of 10. MAST picked up my allergies to cats, dust mites, molds, and pollens, but faltered slightly on foods, correctly pinpointing corn and eggs, while missing wheat. No skin test or in vitro test to date, however, claims to be wholly accurate for foods.

"The ideal procedure," says Clyde Thom, a nuclear engineer/ biochemist who does testing for five Northern California allergists, "is to use the prick test or RAST as a screen in connection with the medical history to give some idea where to start. Then I follow up with intradermals using serial endpoint titration."

Serial titration, also called serial dilution, involves giving the patient various strengths of the allergen until there's little or no reaction. That strength is then used as the starting dose for immunotherapy.

As to which test is superior, Dr. O'Connell states, "Skin tests and RAST are very comparable. Both are 90 percent reliable and effective as diagnostic tools."

Nevertheless, the American Academy of Allergy and Immunology (AAA&I) warns that both skin and RAST testing are open to abuse—most commonly, unwarranted immunotherapy for persons with weakly positive test results and no evidence of allergic disease.

TESTS TO QUESTION

With such a vast market of potential users, experimental tests are bound to proliferate. Some of the following have both doctors and patients who swear by their efficacy. None, however, has met the tough standards required by the AAA&I's board of directors, who have submitted them to intensive review.

Cytotoxic

This blood test claims to determine food, inhalant, and chemical allergies by noting the action of specific allergens on white blood cells. Clinical trials have not shown this method to be effective.

Intradermal Provocation

Diluted allergens are injected beneath the skin in sufficient quantity to elicit (provoke) symptoms. Then, a weaker or stronger dilution of the allergen is injected to relieve (neutralize) symptoms. That dilution is used to establish treatment dosage. (See Chapter 16).

Sublingual Provocation

Using the same provocation-neutralization theory, drops of the diluted allergens are squirted under the tongue. Double-blind studies of provocation-neutralization tests showed no difference in results between placebos and extracts.

This is not to say that these methods don't work, only that they are as yet unproven.

CHAPTER 6

THE BEST MEDICINE

The three basic steps in treating allergy are (1) avoidance, (2) medication, and (3) immunotherapy. Avoidance is the preferred method because it both relieves symptoms and eliminates the cause. In most cases of allergy to foods, drugs, pets, and fabrics, it's the only treatment necessary.

When avoidance isn't possible, medications can help. The most frequently used drugs for treating allergy are antihistamines, which act to block the release of histamine from the mast cells, thus stopping or diminishing symptoms. A major improvement in recent years has been the new breed of antihistamines that causes less drowsiness. Corticosteroid nasal sprays are another new therapy, but with more potential side effects.

Medication plays a vital part in allergy relief, especially when a severe reaction strikes. Then it can literally save your life.

ANTIHISTAMINES—OVER THE COUNTER

Many former prescription drugs are now available over the counter (OTC) in the form of pills, nasal sprays, and eye drops. Americans spend approximately $1.5 billion a year on the growing arsenal of OTC medications and often try them before seeing a doctor.

Be wary of OTC drugs. Buy and use them with as much care and caution as you would a prescribed medication. According to *Consumer Reports on Health*, one in three persons who takes OTC antihistamines also takes other drugs at the same time.

If you know your pharmacist, ask him or her to enter the medication, as well as any drug allergies you may have, in the pharmacy's computer. It should warn about potential drug interactions and possible allergic reactions.

A consumers' book on medicines is an excellent resource. It lists everything you need to know about each drug, including purpose, duration, possible side effects, dosages, and interactions to avoid. (*The Complete Drug Reference* is available in most libraries or from Consumer Reports Books. Send $39.95 to Box 10637, Des Moines, IA 50336, or call 515-237-4903.)

If you're allergic to aspirin, for example, you would need to know that Alka-Seltzer Plus Nighttime Cold contains aspirin, or that ibuprofen (Advil, Motrin-IB) and naproxen (Aleve) can trigger reactions in aspirin-sensitive persons.

Also, alcohol in cough syrups could combine with antihistamines to cause extreme drowsiness, and you could be getting a double dose of antihistamines when you take them with Alka Seltzer Plus Cold, Contac Severe Cold Formula, or sleeping aids Nytol and Sominex—all of which contain antihistamines.

Another point to remember is that antihistamines only help allergies. If you have some other condition, such as sinusitis, antihistamines can prolong the infection by drying out the sinuses and preventing drainage.

Ask your physician for advice before using any OTC drug you haven't used before. And always, *read the package insert or label carefully and follow instructions.*

Here's what to look for:

• What the product does (it should say "allergy relief" or similar words).

• List of active ingredients (are you allergic to any ingredients? Are you taking another drug with the same ingredient and getting a double dose?).

- Instructions for use (dosage; when and how to take it).
- How the drug should be stored.
- Drug interaction precautions (does the drug interact with other medication or with any food or beverage?).
- Tamper-prevention safeguards (don't take any package that shows cuts, tears, or the slightest imperfection).
- Expiration date (never use an outdated drug).
- Warnings (specific medical conditions, including pregnancy, that might preclude taking the drug; possible side effects; when to stop using the product).

Most OTC allergy drugs contain both an antihistamine, to block the action of histamine, and a decongestant to "unstuff" your nose. Some familiar brand-name products that contain both medications are Allerest, Actifed, Dimetapp, and Tavist-D. Tavist-1, Dimetane, Benadryl 25, and Chlor-Trimeton contain only antihistamine; Actifed Allergy, Sudafed, Propagest, and Efidac/24 contain only a decongestant; Tylenol Allergy Sinus contains both, plus a pain reliever.

OTC medications can offer temporary relief, but they do have side effects. Antihistamines can cause dry mouth and drowsiness along with impaired visual, mental, and motor skills. Decongestants tend to wake you up and can cause irritability and insomnia. Reactions vary so widely, you may want to try half a pill first to determine its effects.

Timing can be crucial to getting results. If you're visiting Aunt Ella and her four cats, for instance, or you're en route to a hayride during pollen season, plan ahead. Take antihistamines for three to four days in advance to build up blood levels. If that's not possible, take a tablet at least 30 minutes before the anticipated exposure. Relief usually begins within half an hour and peaks at 45–60 minutes. Remember: One pill taken early can prevent the need for many pills later.

Your body may eventually build up a tolerance to the drug so that it's no longer effective. When that happens, a switch to another drug may help, or it may be time to go back to your doctor.

ANTIHISTAMINES—DOCTOR-PRESCRIBED

Antihistamines fall into several different groups with varying properties. If one type of pill doesn't work for you, another type might. The only way to know if an antihistamine will help you is to try it.

The newer nonsedating antihistamines require a prescription and cost more, but have fewer side effects than "first-generation" antihistamines, and are definitely the agents of choice. Examples are loratadine (Claritin), terfenadine (Seldane), and astemizole (Hismanal). They have proven to be effective and well tolerated, although their safety in pregnancy has not been absolutely determined.

In May of 1994, Reuters news service carried a story linking several of the new antihistamines to cancer growth in mice. The National Cancer Institute promptly responded that the known benefits of the drugs outweighed the known harm, and an FDA advisory committee found it "unlikely that these drugs produce tumors in humans." The furor quickly died down.

When your doctor prescribes an antihistamine, be prepared to ask some questions:

- What will this drug do for me?

- What's the best way to take it? (With fruit juice? With meals?)

- What's the best time to take it?

- How many times a day can I take it?

- Should I take it even if I'm not having symptoms?

- What foods, drinks, or activities should I avoid when I take it? (Alcohol and tranquilizers increase the sedative effects.)

- Will it interact with other medication I'm taking?

- What are the possible side effects?

- Is a generic equivalent available and appropriate?

Short-acting antihistamines can be taken three to four times a day, as needed, while time-release pills are better suited to chronic use. Most of the newer antihistamines are available in once-daily dosages that take effect within half an hour and last for 24 hours.

NASAL SPRAYS

Over-the-counter nasal sprays afford temporary relief from allergic rhinitis, but if used for more than three days they can cause a "rebound effect" that clogs the nose—exactly the opposite of what you want them to do.

Some patients have luck with old-fashioned saltwater sprays. You can buy such products as AYR Saline Nasal Mist, or you can make your own preservative-free solution. Add one teaspoon salt and a pinch of baking soda to a pint of warm water and stir thoroughly. Squirt a half-dropperful into each nostril morning and night. Try for one or two weeks before looking for results. (See Chapter 13 for more details.)

Prescription sprays include cromolyn sodium (Nasalcrom), which has no significant side effects and can prevent mild hay fever symptoms for some people. The drawback is that it must be started 24–36 hours in advance and used 4–6 times a day during allergen exposure. It does not provide relief once symptoms have occurred. Cromolyn is also available in eye drops (Opticrom) for treating allergic conjunctivitis.

Corticosteroid (CCS) nasal sprays such as beclomethasone (Beconase AQ, Vancenase AQ), flunisolide (Nasalide), and triamcinolone (Nasacort, Azmacort) are more effective at reducing mucus flow and shrinking inflamed tissues than cromolyn. Unlike steroid pills, which affect the whole system, topical (affecting only one location or organ) steroids are activated only in the nose and have less effect on the adrenal glands and the rest of the body.

They can, however, cause mouth and throat irritations, reactions that can be reduced by rinsing thoroughly with water after each inhalation. (See Chapter 13 for asthma medication.)

EMERGENCY MEDICATION

Anaphylaxis, as explained earlier, is a violent allergic reaction characterized by a sudden drop in blood pressure and swollen air passages that make breathing difficult. If not treated immediately, breathing becomes impossible. Patients who have had this terrifying experience know they must carry an ANA-kit that contains oral antihistamines, alcohol swabs, and a medication-filled syringe designed for self-use.

The injector delivers a premeasured dose of epinephrine (also called adrenaline), a powerful hormone that dilates the airways, raises blood pressure, and halts symptoms long enough for the patient to get to a medical facility. Best known of the self-injectors is the EpiPen, a boon to anyone who hates needles. The user simply removes the gray safety cap, presses the unit firmly to the outer thigh, and holds it in place several seconds. The mechanism injects the drug automatically.

A new product, the EpiPen trainer, looks and works like the regular model, but without the needle or the medicine. It serves as a practice tool to teach you or your child how to use and feel comfortable with the injector.

DON'T LEAVE HOME WITHOUT IT

People who know they're hypersensitive can arm themselves with medication, but what about those who have never had an anaphylactic reaction?

Ann S., a 32-year-old law student, bought some "high energy bee pollen" pills at the health food store, took one, and suddenly began to feel light-headed. Her heart started to race, and her throat swelled until it almost shut off her air-way. Fortunately, her husband rushed her to a hospital where she was given oxygen, epinephrine, and intravenous fluids—just in time.

Careful testing later revealed she had an exquisite sensitivity to bee venom. Today she carries antihistamine pills and an EpiPen and wears a Medic Alert bracelet engraved with critical facts about her condition.

If you've ever had severe allergy or an asthma attack, you should always carry Medic Alert identification. This is particularly true if you're allergic to any medication. Medic Alert's 24-hour hot-line number (800-432-5378) supplies details of your medical history. (See Appendix C.)

A last word on anaphylaxis: It's extremely rare. Chances are you'll never have to worry.

CHAPTER 7

IMMUNOTHERAPY— CALLING THE SHOTS

Doug C., a star high school athlete, was unlucky enough to be allergic to grass pollen—the kind that floats over football fields.

Avoidance was impossible; medication helped only slightly. In desperation, he went to see an allergist. Relief was neither immediate nor total, but after five months of injections Doug found that he could play football almost an hour longer before starting to sneeze.

Eager to further improve his condition, he learned as much as he could about allergy. The concept of a tolerance threshold made sense, and the more he cut down his exposure to other allergens, the better he began to feel. A year later, the combination of shots, avoidance, and occasional medication gave him enough confidence to accept a football scholarship to an Ivy League college.

Treatment has many success stories, from moderate to major. The advantages of immunotherapy are that it attacks the cause, not the symptoms, has a long safety record, and uses no drugs. But it also has failures and should not be considered a cure. Best results come from persons with:

- Clear-cut IgE-mediated allergies to specific substances.
- Poor or inadequate response to medication.

- Symptoms that have persisted over several seasons or throughout the year.

WHAT TO EXPECT

Immunotherapy aims to desensitize you by injecting you with gradually increasing doses of the substances to which you're allergic. When you reach maximum tolerance, that is, when you begin to show a slight reaction, the increases stop and the dosage is maintained at that level.

In the bloodstream, the injected allergen causes stepped-up production of IgG, the antibody that blocks the action of IgE. You then become partially or wholly desensitized to a particular allergen.

This building up of immunity can take from 3 to 12 months, and sometimes must be continued for several years or longer until you're free of symptoms or able to control them with medication. If symptoms recur, shots can be restarted, but for 50 percent of patients results last indefinitely.

From your point of view, immunotherapy is as easy as taking a weekly or monthly shot in the arm. Allergists will ask you to wait in the office 15–30 minutes to be sure you won't have a bad reaction. For a mild local reaction, you can:

- Take aspirin, acetaminophen (Tylenol, Anacin-3), ibuprofen (Advil, Nuprin, Motrin), or naproxen sodium (Aleve) if the area is sore.
- Take an antihistamine for itching and redness.
- Apply ice if it's swollen.

Some doctors allow you to inject yourself, a great convenience when getting to the office is difficult, or early in treatment when shots may be needed two or more times a week. If there's no improvement at all after 3 to 6 months, stop the shots and look for other ways to find relief.

Allergists who champion immunotherapy claim to see positive results in 80 percent of their patients.

A word of caution: Taking beta-blockers, such as propranolol (Inderal) or nadolol (Corgard), with immunotherapy may be hazardous to your health. The combination can cause spasms of the respiratory passages and lead to breathing difficulty.

WHICH EXTRACTS WORK

An FDA panel of allergy experts recently found that 1,500 extracts on the market were effective for skin tests, but not necessarily for treatment. All standardized extracts used for immunotherapy got high marks, others got question marks. Here's the current status:

- *Insects and bee stings.* The FDA has standardized six insect venoms: yellow hornet, wasp, honeybee, white-faced hornet, yellow jacket, and mixed vespid (wasp mixture). Venom immunotherapy is considered 97 percent effective.

- *Ragweed.* Short ragweed is standardized, and 85 percent of patients in double-blind studies showed improvement.

- *Pollen.* Eight grass pollens are standardized: orchard grass, perennial rye, timothy grass, redtop grass, Kentucky bluegrass, Bermuda grass, meadow fescue, and sweet vernal. Studies show that grass pollen shots are effective.

- *House dust.* Two house dust mites are standardized, but not the dust itself. Some allergists say each person's dust is unique, so that it's impossible to get good results. Others claim treatment works well.

- *Cat.* Two cat extracts are standardized: cat pelt that contains skin cells or dander, and cat hair that's been shaved off the pelt. Until recently, researchers thought the problem was mainly dander. Now they know it's also the saliva cats use while grooming. According to a Swedish study, people with moderate exposure were able to tolerate 11 times more cat allergen after a year of injections. If you're around cats all day, however, shots probably won't help.

- *Dog.* Studies are inconclusive, but many allergists feel that shots work well.

- *Molds.* Crude preparations of arbitrarily chosen fungi may or may not help. Some satisfactory results have been obtained after many months of treatment, but the shots usually cause skin irritations.

- *Poison oak and ivy.* No effective extracts are available.

- *Foods.* No food extracts are standardized at this time. FDA regulatory coordinator Susie Sensabaugh says, "Food extracts don't necessarily immunize. We recommend avoidance." So do most doctors. Of all the allergens used in testing and treatment, food extracts are the most likely to provoke a severe reaction.

RUSH IMMUNOTHERAPY

A speeded-up version, "rush immunotherapy," is performed when a person suddenly needs protection from an anticipated exposure and does not have time for gradual desensitization.

Because of increased risks of a reaction, the patient is hospitalized for constant monitoring, and literally rushed through the first phases. Instead of daily or weekly shots, steadily stronger doses of extract are given every 1–2 hours for a period of 5–10 days. Once the maintenance dose is reached, the patient goes on a schedule similar to conventional treatment.

Warning: This is still an experimental therapy.

ORAL IMMUNOTHERAPY

Oral immunotherapy refers to building immunity by giving patients gradually increased quantities of extracts to drink. Still in research, oral immunotherapy should be distinguished from drops that are squirted beneath the tongue to deliver a maintenance or neutralizing dosage.

"So far, the most encouraging results have been with oral immunotherapy," says the Mayo School of Medicine's Dr. Edward O'Connell. "A number of doctors use sublingual drop therapy, and we get testimonials day in, day out, about its effectiveness. I don't scoff at that at all. But when compared with a placebo, the results are inconclusive."

PART III

WHAT YOU CAN DO

You may never have starred on stage or screen but you definitely play the leading role in your allergy treatment. The part calls for you to be observant and analytical at all times and to take steps to separate yourself from as many allergens as possible.

Here are three ways to do that:

- Clean up your surroundings.

- Learn about your skin. Much can be done to prevent insect stings, eczema, hives, and rashes.

- Study your reaction to foods. Changing your diet is one of the easiest ways to help manage your symptoms.

CHAPTER 8

ALLERGY-PROOF YOUR ENVIRONMENT

Outdoor allergens are almost impossible to control. In your home, however, you rule the atmosphere. The cleaner the air you breathe, and the more dust, pollens, molds, and dander you can banish from your indoor environment, the better your chances of getting good results from pills, sprays, or shots. Your eventual goal is to live and work in settings so free of irritants and allergens that you won't need any medication.

CLEANING HOUSE

Dust reduction is your main priority. Begin in the bedroom, because it's where adults spend one-third of their time and children spend half of their time. It's also home to the greatest number of dust mites. Once you've done the bedroom, apply the same principles to the rest of the house, including closets.

The Bed

Not a pretty picture, but do you realize that thousands of tiny dust mites share your bed and bedding every night? If you weren't so hospitable, they'd starve—and that's exactly what you want to happen. The little beasties can't crawl through plastic, so encase your mattress and box spring in airtight zippered covers, then apply tape over the zippers. (See Appendix D for where to buy products.) The bed should be made of wood or metal.

Avoid wool, down, feather, kapok, and (mold-attracting) foam rubber products. Polyester, linens, or cottons are fine for most people. Blankets, sheets, and pillow cases should be machine-washed in very hot water (130° F.) every 7–14 days.

Eliminate such dust collectors as quilts and comforters, and in general, keep your bed simple. Canopies, padded headboards, bunk beds and ruffles are far too hospitable to mites.

The Floor

New carpet loses its strong chemical odor over time, but as it ages, it becomes a haven for microorganisms—dust mites, mold spores, animal dander, and the like. A recent University of Virginia study found that carpets accumulate allergens at 100 times the rate of a bare floor.

If possible, carpets should be replaced. The ideal nonallergenic floor is a hardwood, tile, or vinyl surface that can be cleaned with a wet mop—twice a week, at least—and covered with small washable rugs. Don't use brooms; they stir up too much dust.

If carpets cannot be removed, keep pets off them as much as possible. Vacuum once a week, or better yet, have someone else do the vacuuming. Stay out of the room for at least half an hour until the dust settles.

The best vacuum to buy is a tank-type with strong suction and an extension on the hose so that the canister can sit outside the room during vacuuming. Dust-filtering bags are available from allergy supply companies for about $11 a set, but leave the task of changing them to someone else.

Some vacuum cleaners come equipped with HEPA (high-efficiency particulate-arresting) filters specially designed to collect fine particles. *Consumer Reports* studied vacuum cleaners in

1993 and reported: "People with allergies might look to the Nilfisk GS 90 canister, $645. It was so effective at filtering dust particles that it actually cleaned the air slightly while we tested. Several less expensive models—primarily soft-bag uprights—also received high scores for filtration." (See Appendix D.)

Have your carpets steam-cleaned regularly at the hottest possible temperature. Mites only meet their maker at 130° F. or higher. Don't shampoo your rugs. Leftover soap produces dust, and moisture invites molds.

Check with your doctor or pharmacist before using an acaracide, a mite-killing product. Most release chemical irritants such as benzyl benzoate into the air.

The Windows

Roll-down shades and unlined washable curtains are preferable to dust-catching blinds and draperies. Keep windows closed during pollen season and at peak pollen hours, usually 5 A.M. to 10 A.M. Use central or room air conditioning switched to the "Recycle" or "Recirculate" setting. Air conditioners are great pollen traps, so clean them and change filters scrupulously.

The Bathroom

Prevent molds from growing by wiping down shower curtains, walls, tub, toilet, tile, and all damp areas with a mixture of ½ cup bleach to 1 gallon of water at least once a month. Four times a year use Zephiran (benzalkonium chloride), one fluid ounce to a gallon of water, to further inhibit mold growth. Allow plenty of ventilation, and let surfaces air-dry—or better yet, install an exhaust fan.

The Kitchen

Don't allow food to spoil, but if it does, discard it immediately, then wash and dry receptacles thoroughly. Use a fan or open the windows to remove excess steam when cooking. Look out for mold on cutting boards and sponges, in sink and disposer stoppers, refrigerator gaskets and drip pans, washing machines, garbage containers, and places where fresh food is stored.

Watch for dust and mildew atop, behind, and under sinks, stoves, refrigerators, and other hard-to-reach places.

All Rooms

Bare is beautiful. The fewer objects lying around, the better. Books, magazines, light fixtures, shelves of knickknacks, TV sets, even clothes collect dust. Move small objects to drawers and cabinets and keep all garments in clean closets with closed doors. If you must dust the room yourself, use damp rather than dry dusting, and wear a face mask.

Painted walls are preferable to wallpaper because the flour in wallpaper paste has a high content of mold spores. So do fabric hangings and tapestries. If practical, replace upholstered chairs and sofas with canvas, metal, plastic, or simple wood furniture.

Decorative pillows and stuffed animals attract dust. One mother tells her daughter she's taking her teddy bear for a ride, then pops him into the dryer for a half-hour spin at high heat. An alternative is to put Teddy in an airtight plastic bag and place him in the freezer for a full two to three days. It takes that long for the cold temperature to kill the mites, although it doesn't remove their debris. A third possibility is to cut open the toy, replace the stuffing with old nylon stockings or polyester fill, and sew up the seam.

Many doctors recommend air conditioners to reduce humidity and discourage molds and mites, which need at least 50 percent humidity to survive. Ideal humidity levels should be 30–40 percent. Cover vents tightly with HEPA or electrostatic air filters, and clean or change the filters regularly. Bedroom air conditioners are best operated at night when pollen levels are lowest. (Some allergists question the use of air conditioners to reduce molds, so check with your doctor before making a purchase.)

Other steps you can take to reduce molds:

- Use the stove vent while cooking.
- Keep a 75-watt bulb burning in closets to keep them dry.
- Keep storage rooms, attics, and basements clean and dry.
- Install exhaust fans in bathrooms.
- Be sure clothing, linens, luggage, garden supplies, and outdoor play equipment are not put away soiled or damp.

High room temperatures (about 70° F.) and dehumidifiers can also help keep the air dry, particularly in moist climates. Empty and clean your dehumidifier every other day.

HUMIDIFIERS

For some people, extremely dry air can trigger asthma and nasal congestion and make irritated nasal membranes more susceptible to assaults by allergens and irritants. In this case, ideal humidity levels would be higher, around 40–60 percent.

If you're not allergic to molds and mites, your doctor may recommend a humidifier to relieve the discomfort of dry eyes, nose, lips, mouth, and/or skin. These symptoms particularly plague people who live in warm or desert climates.

Humidifiers can be helpful in keeping the air moist and your airways well-hydrated, but if the tanks are not cleaned religiously, the accumulated bacteria can cause an inflammation known as "humidifier lung."

Your daily care routine should follow these steps:

1. Empty the humidifier tank and wash carefully with hot, soapy water. Rinse under faucet and fill to appropriate level with tap (or preferably distilled) water.

2. After use, clean tank again, add 2 cups of white vinegar and enough water to enable the machine to create vapor. Run 30 minutes in a well-ventilated area, then rinse again.

3. Fill with water, run for 3 minutes, rinse twice. Keep dry until next usage.

Ultrasonic humidifiers should be used with caution. Some spew into the air minerals that could irritate the lungs.

AIR CLEANERS

Many doctors recommend indoor air-cleaning devices for patients with respiratory problems. Good models, designed to clean an entire room, are available for $175 and up. Some companies will allow you to rent or lease one on a trial basis.

The efficiency of these machines has long been in dispute. Some say they're wonderful, others insist they're worthless. Part of the answer depends on the weight of the airborne particles and how long they stay in the air.

Animal dander, for instance, is tiny and light and floats for a long time. Larger specks such as pollens or dust mite particles drop quickly. Within 10 minutes, 95 percent of pollens fall from the air spontaneously. Air cleaners are only effective on those particles still in the air.

There are two main types of air cleaners:

Mechanical filters

These use layers of densely packed fibers to trap the particles as the air passes through. The most effective mechanical filter, the HEPA (high-efficiency particulate-arresting), collects 95–99.97 percent of the small particles.

Consumer Reports Buying Guide of 1994 gives high ratings to the Enviracaire EV-35B model ($300) and the Austin Air Sierra HEPA PFA-80-AC by Healthmate ($395).

Electronic Devices

These charge the particles, then draw them in by attraction to a plate carrying the opposite charge. The electrostatic precipitator is highly recommended, but requires frequent cleaning. Otherwise it can produce ozone which may irritate the airways.

Consumer Reports recommends the Friedrich C90, $439. "It was by far the most effective in our tests. The best tabletop unit we tested was the Pollenex 1850, $60. But the annual electricity cost, $80, makes it a poor value. The Trion Super Clean II, $129, didn't perform as well, but may be a better choice . . . (with) annual operating costs around $52."

In short, air cleaners can remove pollens, dander, spores, smoke, and dust, but never completely eliminate gases, tobacco odors, viruses, bacteria, or pollutants that constantly enter the house from outside.

An air cleaner should be set in the middle of a closed room but not on a carpet where it can stir up settled dust. Run it on high after vacuuming and after pets, smokers, or heavy perfume-wearers have been present. (If pets live in other parts of the house, keep their litter boxes meticulously clean.)

For more home protection, equip your heating outlets with a dust filter that you clean or change once a month. Use small electric heaters whenever possible, and avoid burning wood in the fireplace. The smoke adds mold, insect debris, pollen, and dust particles to the air.

PLANTS

Potted plants increase indoor humidity and release mold spores and pollen. Wicker products and Christmas trees can also contribute to problems.

But don't toss out that cymbidium just yet. According to William C. Wolverton, Ph.D., an environmental scientist recently retired from the National Aeronautics and Space Administration (NASA), certain plants can "swallow" allergens and pollutants, cleaning and revitalizing indoor air.

Dr. Wolverton believes that low-light-requiring plants work their magic by metabolizing pollutants drawn in through their leaves and roots. They also, he claims, emit a substance that reduces airborne levels of mold spores and bacteria.

Here are some plants he's tested, and the pollutants they absorb best:

- *Anthurium:* ammonia, xylene
- *Boston fern:* formaldehyde
- *Chrysanthemum:* benzene, formaldehyde
- *Devil's ivy:* benzene, carbon monoxide
- *Dwarf date palm:* ammonia, formaldehyde, xylene
- *Elephant ear philodendron:* benzene, carbon monoxide
- *English ivy:* benzene
- *Ficus benjamina:* formaldehyde, ammonia, xylene
- *Orchid:* acetone, methyl alcohol, ethyl acetate
- *Peace lily:* benzene, formaldehyde
- *Yellow tulip:* formaldehyde, ammonia, xylene

Dr. Wolverton foresees the day when high-rise apartments and office towers will be filled with plants that will totally cleanse and recycle their air. The Environmental Protection Agency is interested, but so far does not support the scientist's claims.

ALLERGENS ON THE JOB

Does working making you sick? It could. Almost every job or occupation can be linked to some form of allergy, particularly respiratory. Photographers, plumbers, and all who work near moisture are in constant contact with molds; gardeners, florists, and athletes are particularly subject to pollens; veterinarians, jockeys, and farm hands can build up reactions to animal dander; and they're all exposed to dust.

Office and factory workers often develop sensitivities to chemicals (see Chapters 15–18), which are different from toxic reactions. When a highway accident releases clouds of chemical fumes and hundreds of people are treated for symptoms, that's a toxic reaction. When a minute quantity of that same chemical causes symptoms in one person and doesn't affect anyone else, that's allergy.

Surprisingly, the office environment today is more conducive to good health than it was 10 years ago. There are many reasons, including:

- Fewer people smoke indoors.

- The frenzy of the mid-1970s to energy-seal buildings has somewhat diminished; new buildings are not quite as airtight as before, and not recirculating as much dusty and polluted air.

- People are back to opening windows if outdoor pollution permits.

- Office equipment has been improved to give off fewer fumes.

- There is greater awareness of indoor air contaminants, which cause "sick building" syndrome (see Chapter 17), and less use of strong perfumes, cleaning solvents, toxic paints, varnishes, glues, and adhesives.

Diagnosing workplace allergy, however, can be a challenge. Reactions are sometimes delayed, sometimes triggered by a combination of substances, sometimes caused by a relatively unknown allergen.

Here's where you play detective again. Observe, keep records, persevere for as long as it takes to discover the cause of your problem.

Your symptoms are probably work-related if:

- They occur only on the job.

- You can relate them to a time, a smell, an object such as a copier, or a location in the workplace.

- They diminish on weekends.

- They disappear on vacations.

- Some co-workers have similar symptoms.

Employers have a legal responsibility to ensure healthful working conditions and to provide you with whatever protective gear you need—masks, gloves, safety glasses, coveralls. Be sure to request any supplies you think would help, as well as filters, traps, fans, or air cleaners. If strong janitorial solvents pervade the area, speak to your employer about using substitute products.

Some employers may be reluctant to cooperate. In this case, check your phone book for the nearest state or federal office of the Occupational Safety and Health Administration (OSHA), and consider making a complaint. The law ensures that your name will be kept confidential.

At the same time, see your doctor and proceed as you would with any allergy: avoid, diagnose, treat.

TIPS FOR TRAVEL

What may seem obvious, often is not. To ensure a healthy vacation, pick a destination as free of your particular allergens as possible. Skip the primitive countries with their dusty ruins and moldy caves. Head for beaches and mountains (over 5,000 feet) where the air is cleanest. Take along whatever medications you may need, and always wear your Medic Alert dogtag or bracelet.

Car travel should be in a clean, air-conditioned vehicle free of dust, pet dander, and cigarette smoke. Keep windows closed and try to drive along a coast highway rather than an inland route. Park away from trees so that pollen won't collect in the intake vents or on the surface of your car.

If you're flying, taking an antihistamine/decongestant half an hour before you board will keep your nasal passages clear and spare you some of the discomfort of pressure changes. Swallowing saliva or chewing gum on takeoff and landing will also help.

Ocean vessels, especially in warm climates, are ideal for persons sensitive to airborne allergens. Unless it's a moldy old freighter, the more time you spend at sea, on the deck, the better you'll feel.

Once you get to your destination, avoid "quaint" resorts with wood-buring fireplaces and overstuffed furniture; cheap lodgings liable to have moldy bathrooms (especially in the tropics); and friends' homes where you have no control of your surroundings.

Instead, choose a clean, modern, smoke-free hotel where you can ask the maid to go easy on the disinfectant, turn up the heat, have your bedding changed frequently, and call the desk when anything goes wrong.

CHAPTER 9

SAVING YOUR SKIN

R andy Z., a high school senior, thought it would be cool to get his left ear pierced for graduation. Three days after the procedure, however, his earlobe began to swell and itch.

"It's God's way of telling you that real men don't wear earrings," his father insisted. His mother, a nurse, suspected a more earthly explanation and urged Randy to remove the small metal pin that kept the hole in his ear open. She coated it with clear nail polish to act as a barrier between skin and metal, then told him to try again.

Randy was delighted. Now he could wear his badge of coolness with no discomfort. But alas, the pin was made of a nickel alloy that sensitized him to nickel all over his body. Forced to change his metal eyeglass frames for plastic ones, and no longer able to wear his watchband or work with his favorite garden tools, he wondered: Was it worth it?

If only we could know in advance that piercing an ear would trigger a nickel allergy, petting a cat would elicit a rash, or eating shrimps would cause hives, we'd probably think twice before doing any of those things. But unfortunately, first-time allergies aren't preventable. We have no way of knowing we're susceptible until we start getting symptoms.

Randy's sore ear would be classified as contact dermatitis, a skin rash caused by physical contact. When it's nonallergic, it can be as simple as red, itchy hands irritated by a soap or detergent. The reaction is superficial and does not involve the immune system. Skin irritations are far more common than allergic reactions.

Allergic contact dermatitis (ACD) can be an acute or chronic skin eruption triggered by cosmetics, fragrances, dyes, fabrics, metals, rubber, plants, pet saliva, chemicals, and so on. The distinction between allergy and irritation doesn't always matter. If latex gloves make your hands itch, don't wear them.

The good news is that your skin is right there in front of you, visible and tangible. You can see, smell, and touch what's going on. With care and astute observations, contact skin allergies can be among the easiest ailments to heal.

ECZEMA

Mary Rose was nine when she first noticed a dry, cracking rash on her hands. Her father, a surgeon, said it was "just eczema" and gave her antihistamine pills to relieve the itching.

A week later, the rash flared so dramatically that her mother took her to an allergist. Subsequent probing and testing showed that Mary Rose was allergic to milk—and also to the antihistamines. The treatment was making her worse! When she stopped the pills and went on a milk-free diet, her rash subsided.

Eczema or atopic dermatitis (AD) follows no format or formula. It can appear at any age, although it's most prevalent in babies and children. It can affect any area of the body but usually starts on the face or over elbows and knees in babies. About 85 percent of infant eczema cases clear spontaneously during childhood.

Adults are more likely to find patches on the arms, legs, feet, scalp, behind the ears, and especially on the hands.

If you suspect you have eczema, take these steps:

- Check with your doctor to rule out possible causes for the rash other than allergy.
- Be on the lookout for all irritants and substances, including

foods that seem to cause burning, itching, redness, or dryness.

- Prevent skin dryness. Bathe or lubricate your skin once or twice a day. Use warm (not hot) water, minimal soap, and no bubble bath (whch may contain irritants).

- Moisturize with nonirritant cream, vegetable oil, or petroleum jelly (Vaseline) within three minutes after bathing and as often as necessary to keep skin from becoming scaly. (Moisturizers work best on wet skin.)

- Avoid lotions that contain water and alcohol; they have a drying effect. Greasy ointments are better absorbed than creams.

- Minimize contact with household cleaners, dyes, chemicals, body care goods, fragrances, cosmetics, and products such as jewelry or watchbands that might contain nickel. Lanolin, an oil obtained from sheep, and Quarternium-15, a preservative in shampoos and lotions, are also frequent sensitizers.

- Wear gloves for dishwashing and household chores, but be wary of latex, which often causes irritations.

- For mild itching, ask your doctor or pharmacist for an OTC anti-itch medication. "Calamine doesn't do much," says dermatologist Dr. John H. Epstein. "If the rash is weeping, you can use cool water compresses."

- Use medication immediately after a bath or a soak to increase absorption.

- Wear loose, lightweight cotton clothing; no heavy wools or synthetics.

- Change or rotate the brand of laundry detergent you use.

- Trim your nails. Scratching can lead to infection.

- Avoid extremes or rapid changes of temperature.

- Avoid strenuous activity or exercise. Sweat can aggravate the rash.

- Recognize and reduce stress. It leads to itching.

If eczema is confirmed, your doctor may suggest an OTC topical corticoid ointment, or a stronger, prescription corticosteroid (CCS) cream. These are potent drugs; 1.4 percent of patients become allergic to the creams and ointments themselves.

Follow instructions: apply sparingly, rub in well, and don't use medication prescribed for one rash on the next skin irritation. Short-term use should cause no problems, but long-term use of topical steroids can cause thinning of the skin and easy bruising.

HIVES

Urticaria is the medical term for hives, the itchy wheals that look like mosquito bites. *Angioedema* refers to giant hives associated with swelling of other parts of the body, especially around the eyes and lips. *Dermographism* is a form of hives that develops when the skin is rubbed, stroked, or pressured.

Hives usually appear shortly after exposure to an allergen and can show up anywhere on the skin. They may be harmless and disappear within hours, or they may be an early symptom of anaphylaxis. Some likely triggers are:

- Foods—mainly berries, seafood, nuts, tomatoes, eggs, and wheat
- Food additives, especially dyes and preservatives.
- Drugs or medication, including aspirin and penicillin
- Insect bites or stings.
- Any number of substances including fabrics and detergents (although hives from contact reactions are rare).
- Physical stimuli such as a cold swimming pool or a hot shower, sudden temperature changes, sunlight, exercise, vigorous toweling after bathing, or tight clothing.
- Cold weather. (If you suspect a cold allergy and want to test yourself, wrap an ice cube in plastic and hold it to your skin

for 30–60 seconds. A raised welt indicates a positive reaction.)

- Chemical fumes.
- Stress and anxiety.

Treat hives with oral antihistamines around the clock, anti-itch lotion, if necessary, and avoid all suspected allergens. If the welts don't vanish in 48 hours, see your doctor.

LEAVES OF THREE, TURN AND FLEE

The most notorious triggers of ACD are the three members of the Rhus family of plants. Poison ivy with its clusters of three leaves grows mostly on the East Coast. Poison oak also has three-pronged leaves and is found in the South and on the West Coast. Poison sumac, a fernlike shrub, grows near streams and swampy areas.

As their names indicate, these plants are not user-friendly. Seventy percent of Americans who touch them will react to urushiol, the toxic oil that causes a delayed itching, burning, blistering rash.

Learn to recognize and avoid the Rhus family. Despite many claims, neither oral drops nor injections have proven effective as preventives.

If you're exposed, here's what to do:

1. Immediately wash the affected area with water. According to Dr. Epstein, "The only way applying alcohol will do any good is if you use it within seconds after exposure. Otherwise, take a lukewarm—not hot—shower. Use soap, but don't rub or scrub."

2. Blot yourself dry. Use a clean area of the towel each time, so as not to spread the oil, especially into your eyes.

3. Wash clothes, garden tools, car doors, even pets—anything that may have touched any part of the plant.

4. Relieve mild symptoms with anti-itch medication, an OTC hydrocortisone cream, or a solution of 1 tablespoon vinegar to a gallon of water in a bathtub or on compresses.

5. Take an oral antihistamine.

Contrary to common thought, poison ivy doesn't always go away by itself. Healing depends on how allergic you are to it and how much of it you have. For severe cases, your doctor may advise short-term use of oral steroids.

To destroy poison ivy plants, use a nursery-recommended organic compound or call in a professional. Burying poison ivy contaminates the soil, and burning it produces toxic smoke that can penetrate the eyes, skin, and lungs.

BEAT THE BEES

Insect bites and bee, wasp, or hornet stings are decidedly unpleasant. Your body may react in one of three ways:

1. A small itchy welt appears. It swells at the site and becomes sore and red, but discomfort vanishes in a few hours. The wheal heals by itself and poses no threat to your health.

2. You develop swelling in unrelated parts of the body, a slight cough, confusion, a headache, or other systemic reactions. These symptoms, no matter how mild, should be taken as a serious warning that the next bite or sting could be fatal.

3. Dizziness, flushing, hives, cramping, nausea, coughing, and gasping for breath are signs of a life-threatening reaction that demands immediate medical care. Don't waste a minute!

A few precautions, however, can lower your chances of being a target:

• Wear long sleeves and long pants.

• Wear light-colored clothes. Insects are attracted to bright colors and prints, black, and rough-textured fabrics.

• Avoid flashy jewelry.

- Avoid perfume, hair spray, all scented drugs and cosmetics.
- Don't use insect repellent. The creams and sprays can be toxic to humans.
- Don't walk barefoot through the grass or wear shoes without socks.
- Avoid areas where stinging insects are likely to be found: flower beds and fields, streams and lakes, garbage sites.
- For barbecues and picnics, set out a colorful decoy dish of gooey sweets to draw insects.
- When driving, keep car windows closed.
- If a critter lands on you, try gentle brushing. Swatting and quick jerky movements can provoke a bee to sting. (A sure way to get stung when a bee lands on you is to jump into water.)

Despite all precautions, you may still be irresistible to an insect. If you're stung or bitten, apply an ice pack immediately. Cold reduces swelling and delays the venom getting into the bloodstream. Elevate the affected extremity, and take an oral antihistamine.

If your symptoms seem more complicated or the least bit suspicious, call your doctor.

ALPHA HYDROXY ACIDS (AHA)

The current zeal for face and skin moisturizers containing AHA is not without an occasional price tag. The active ingredient can come from sour milk (lactic acid), sugarcane (glycolic acid), or apples (malic acid), and while safe and effective for the majority of users, it can touch off reactions in sensitive persons. Swollen, tender, or itchy skin may indicate an allergy to the acid or a response to some other ingredient in the cream.

John Bailey, Ph.D., director of the FDA's Office of Cosmetics and Colors, warns that stronger concentrations of AHAs may make the skin's protective barrier permanently thinner, leaving you more susceptible to allergic reactions caused by substances such as makeup and moisturizer.

At the first sign of a problem, stop using the product. Change brands, buy a weaker strength AHA, and try again.

IS "HYPOALLERGENIC" A HYPE?

The easy answer to that question is "Sometimes." FDA Public Affairs Specialist Janet McDonald explains that labels must be accurate in listing ingredients, and ingredients must be safe; however, "There are no regulatory standards on what constitutes 'hypoallergenic.'" The term normally means that the manufacturer feels the product is less likely than others to cause an allergic reaction.

Some manufacturers of "hypoallergenic" or "allergy-free" products simply omit fragrances; others take pains to replace common irritants with safe substitutes. But even those precautions are no guarantee. What's safe for your cousin Irving may not be safe for you.

Don't be fooled by flashy advertising. The law doesn't require cosmetic manufacturers to substantiate performance claims. Question all such terms as "dermatologist-tested," which can mean that a single skin specialist tested the product for allergenic problems. (When? On whom?) Along with "nonirritating," "allergy-tested," and "sensitivity-tested," the labels have little value.

"Unscented" and "fragrance-free" products often use other chemicals to mask odors, and many cosmetics claim to be "natural." These natural ingredients come from plant or animal sources, rather than chemicals in a laboratory, and frequently cause allergies. Lanolin, for example, a common fatlike substance extracted from sheep wool, is highly allergenic.

What claims, then, can you trust? According to the FDA, the following are all classified as cosmetics: skin care creams, lotions, and powders; perfume, makeup, nail polish, polish remover, cuticle softener; hair dyes, conditioners, shampoos;

deodorants, shaving preparations, baby care products; bath oils and bubble bath; mouthwash and toothpaste.

Cosmetic testing is low on the FDA priority list, but major brands with established reputations are generally thought to be safe. Large manufacturers can afford sanitary laboratories, top chemists and researchers, and time to test products before putting them on the market. They don't want customers to suffer negative reactions and they certainly don't want lawsuits.

HOW TO AVOID PROBLEMS WITH COSMETICS

If you do have an allergic response, stop using *all* cosmetics immediately. Call your doctor, who will try to help you determine the cause. Once you've found and eliminated the product(s), follow these suggestions:

- Use all cosmetics in moderation.

- Read labels. Choose products with the simplest, most basic ingredients. (See Chapter 17.)

- Rotate! Buy several different brands of the same product (toothpaste, deodorant, shampoo, lipsticks) and use one on Monday, another Tuesday, and so on. Using the same product day after day increases your chances of developing an allergy to one or more ingredients.

- Don't buy scented products; fragrances are the number one cause of cosmetic allergies. Dyes and preservatives also rank high.

- Use mild, unscented soap or no soap. If your hands are irritated, shower or bathe with protective gloves.

- Use throwaway cotton pads or Q-Tips to apply makeup. Don't use your fingers.

- Wash off all makeup, especially around the eyes, before going to bed.

- Get a good night's sleep. Rest rejuvenates the skin.

CHAPTER 10

FOODS FOR THOUGHT

Francesca P., a fashion model, decided she needed more fiber in her diet. Her usual breakfast was toast and coffee; lunch was a sandwich; dinner was pasta and salad. To this heavy wheat diet she added a daily heaping tablespoon of wheat germ dissolved in water. It tasted terrible, but did its job. Her bowels moved regularly.

Several months into this regime, however, Francesca's hands broke out in a rash that became so bad she had to see a doctor. Hearing about her diet, he was immediately suspicious, and told her to stop eating wheat. Protesting that she had eaten wheat all her life with no problem, she reluctantly stopped— and bingo! her skin soon cleared.

Francesca had brought the allergy on herself by overindulgence. Moderation should always be the rule in eating favorite foods, especially with such a potent allergen as wheat. Unfortunately, Francesca's sensitivity remains. A slice of bread every other day is the most wheat she can presently tolerate without getting eczema.

WHAT IS A FOOD ALLERGY?

A true food allergy, or hypersensitivity, is an abnormal response to a food, triggered by the immune system and involving the production of IgE antibodies.

Food allergies are far less common than most people think. Researchers in Amersham, England, recently surveyed 7,500 households and found that one in five persons—20 percent of the group—believed they had food allergies. When tested, however, fewer than 5 percent showed real sensitivities.

The incidence of true food allergy in America is from 0.1–5 percent, depending on the person's age. Children from birth to age three have the greatest number of food sensitivities. After three, they usually outgrow them, except for shrimp, peanut, and tree nut allergies, which tend to be more severe. Most adult allergies disappear after one to two years of complete avoidance of the offending food.

Almost anyone can develop a food allergy if some or all of these factors are present:

- An inherited tendency to allergy.

- Sufficient time and/or exposure.

- A potent allergen. (Prime suspects are milk, eggs, wheat, peanuts—a legume, not a nut—fruits, corn, soy, nuts, and seafood.)

- A rundown physical condition or illness.

- Stress or emotional trauma.

- Use of mucosal irritants such as aspirin, arthritis medications, or alcohol, which can change the surface of the intestines, allowing more allergens to be absorbed into the system.

HOW THE BODY RESPONDS

Target organs for food allergies can be one or more of the various body systems: gastrointestinal, respiratory, cutaneous (skin), nervous, urinary, and even cardiovascular (heart and blood vessels).

Most allergic food reactions start in the gastrointestinal tract, with bloating, cramps, vomiting, and/or diarrhea. Respiratory

symptoms—sneezing, runny nose, itchy eyes, difficulty breathing—may develop, along with skin eruptions of eczema, hives,
and angioedema.

As always, anaphylaxis is the great danger. It can occur minutes after eating even a tiny particle of food—$\frac{1}{44,000}$ of a peanut,
for example. According to the *Journal of the American Medical Association (JAMA)*, some 1,000 Americans go into anaphylactic
shock every year. About 50 die from it.

Some people get severe symptoms only when they exercise
after eating a particular food (usually celery or shellfish). They
can avoid the problem by not eating for 3–4 hours before a
workout.

Potentially fatal reactions usually start with sweating, itching, and swelling in the tongue and throat, and difficulty breathing. The deadly pattern may progress rapidly or take several
hours. The treatment for anaphylaxis is always the same, no
matter what the cause. If you're susceptible to breathing difficulty or tend to get asthma, always carry an oral antihistamine
and an epinephrine-filled syringe.

ORAL ALLERGY SYNDROME

Suppose you eat beef at lunch with no reaction and drink milk
at dinner with no reaction, but when you eat both at the same
meal, you break out in hives. This is called a cross-reaction because you're responding to the cumulative effects of two members of the same food family.

Cross-reactions occur with nonfood substances, too. For instance, you may be able to eat cantaloupe most of the year, but
when certain grasses begin to pollinate, you find you can't tolerate the melon. This type of allergic reaction, the cross-reacting of
identical allergens present in pollens and fresh foods, is called
oral allergy syndrome or OAS. The symptoms are itching and
swelling of the lips, tongue, mouth, or throat.

Take another example: You're eating a peach in the kitchen
with the windows closed. You decide to sit in the garden, but as

soon as you venture outside, the combination of peach and pollens makes your lips swell.

You'd be right to suspect anaphylaxis because it could be the start of a severe reaction, but if your symptoms stop at the mouth and throat and don't affect your skin, temperature, or breathing, you're probably safe and the swelling should disappear by itself.

If there's the least suspicion that you might be having an anaphylactic reaction, don't wait to find out. Reach for the epinephrine.

HOW TO RECOGNIZE A FOOD ALLERGY

A true food allergy, involving the immune system, differs from a food intolerance—an adverse food reaction that doesn't have an immunologic basis. Differentiating is important in that failing to identify a food allergy may leave you unprepared for a crisis. But how do you tell which is which?

Sometimes it's almost impossible. Ask yourself these questions:

1. Are you allergic to other substances? (If yes, you're more likely to be food-reactive.)

2. Do your reactions occur relatively soon after eating a certain food? (A few minutes to two hours for most allergies, two to six hours for most intolerances.)

3. Do your mouth and throat itch after eating a certain food? (This usually means allergy. If you're sensitive to ragweed, be wary of cantaloupe, honeydew, watermelon, sunflower seeds, cucumbers, and bananas. Some people who experience hives, itching, or wheezing after eating bananas, cherries, water chestnuts, or avocados are also sensitive to condoms, balloons, and latex gloves.)

4. Does your nose run after eating a certain food? (Unless it's hot soup or hot pepper, suspect allergy.)

5. Does your skin break out after eating a certain food? (Skin rashes are a common food allergy symptom.)

6. Do you have abdominal discomfort after eating a certain food? (No clues here. Gastrointestinal upsets such as cramps or diarrhea are common to both allergies and intolerances. When the symptoms are accompanied by a skin rash or a runny nose, however, allergy becomes more likely.)

7. Did others who ate the same food as you did at a particular meal get ill? (If so, the problem may be contamination. Suspect spoiled, unclean, or undercooked fish, meat, poultry, dairy or egg products.)

8. Do certain foods make you feel sad or depressed? (The jury's still debating. Many believe food allergies directly affect emotions. Others disagree.)

Your answers to the preceding questions may give you clues, but not conclusions. In order to better determine what is a food allergy, you need to know what isn't.

FOOD INTOLERANCES

Most food reactions are caused by intolerances rather than allergies. These symptoms, mainly abdominal, occur in response to:

ADDITIVES. The major offenders are preservatives, such as sulfites and benzoate, which can bring on breathing difficulties and asthma. Dyes, especially ponceau (red dye no. 4) and tartrazine (yellow dyes no. 5 and 6) can cause hives and lip swelling, and produce hyperactivity in sensitive children. The flavor enhancer monosodium glutamate (MSG) can induce headaches, asthma, and a tingling and burning in the chest that's sometimes mistaken for a heart attack. (These additives may also be allergens.)

CARBOHYDRATES. Like fiber, some sugars and starches are not completely absorbed in the intestine before reaching the colon.

The symptoms they cause resemble food allergy reactions: abdominal bloating, gas, cramps, and diarrhea.

CONTAMINATION. Insect and rodent parts and excrement, molds, bacteria, parasites, antibiotics, and hepatitis viruses can all adulterate food.

FIBER. Long known to cause stomach distress, fiber often troubles persons who have recently upped their fiber intake. High-fiber foods such as bran, beans, and cruciferous vegetables (broccoli, Brussels sprouts, cabbage, and cauliflower) are well-known gastric offenders.

FRUCTOSE. Fruits and fruit juices are high in this sugar, which sometimes causes abdominal problems. So does sorbitol, the main sweetener in sugar-free gums and candies, also found in apples, peaches, pears, and prunes.

GLUTEN, a protein in wheat. Celiac sprue (intestinal malabsorption) is a sensitivity to gluten, not an allergy, but the treatment is the same: careful avoidance of wheat and all gluten-containing products such as rye, barley, and oats.

HISTAMINE. Certain cheeses, wines, and fish, particularly tuna and mackerel, may have high levels of this compound as a result of bacterial contamination. Symptoms can mimic an allergic reaction.

MILK. Lactose intolerance (lactase deficiency) affects one in ten people, particularly African Americans, Asians, and persons of Mediterranean ancestry. The reaction occurs when an individual lacks sufficient lactase, an enzyme, to digest lactose, the sugar in milk. Bacteria then turns the lactose to gas, causing bloating, abdominal pain, and diarrhea.

High-lactose foods include milk, ice cream, mozzarella, cottage cheese, and other soft cheeses. Yogurt and hard cheeses are lower in lactose. Intolerance to lactose sometimes shows up in adults who haven't had milk for years and suddenly start drinking it to prevent osteoporosis.

Some lactose-intolerant people can manage small amounts of milk. With true milk allergy, *any* consumption of milk or milk products could be dangerous.

PSYCHOLOGICAL TRIGGERS. A sad or traumatic event tied to a particular food can bring a rush of unpleasant sensations that resemble allergy.

RED WINE. It may be the alcohol, which acts to congest the nasal passages, or it may be the phenolic flavonoid compounds from grape skins that give you a headache. Red wine has more of these compounds than white wine.

Symptoms of serious diseases, such as colon cancer, are sometimes mistakenly diagnosed as food allergies. The practice of blaming foods for all sorts of physical ailments is so prevalent that doctors have given it a name: pseudo food allergy. People too busy or too lazy to take the time to discover what's really wrong often jump to the quickest, easiest conclusion.

That's why it's essential to see your doctor. Once he or she has checked your physical condition, ruled out other possibilities, and suspects a true food allergy, you may be asked to keep records of your food intake and symptoms.

DAILY DIARY

Skin and blood tests can offer clues, but the only sure way to discover what's causing your symptoms is to (1) keep a food diary for one to two weeks and (2) test your observations with an elimination diet and oral challenges (the careful reintroduction of foods).

Here are some tips to help you get the most from your diary:

- Carry it in your purse or pocket at all times. It needn't be bulky; a slim notepad will do.
- Write down everything you lick, chew, suck on, or digest, including vitamin pills, medication, chewing gum.
- Be specific. Don't write "chicken salad." Write: "chicken breast (no skin), green onions, celery," and so on.
- Include spices, seasonings, even water. (Tap or bottled? Spring or carbonated?)
- If a prepared or processed food has a long ingredient list, save the label and attach it to your food diary.
- Record all symptoms, no matter how minor they seem.

FOOD DIARY

DATE/TIME OF MEAL

MENU

SYMPTOMS

TIME SYMPTOMS BEGAN

WHAT HAPPENED TO SYMPTOMS (Did they persist, worsen, or disappear?)

At the end of a week, compare good and bad days, and try to spot patterns of response to specific foods.

Some other factors to consider:

1. Did you react to the food every time you ate it? (This could be either an allergy or an intolerance.)

2. Did you react one time and not the next? (This could be for a variety of reasons. See next section.)

3. Did you have wine or any other alcoholic beverage? (Alcohol increases the absorption of food allergens.)

4. Were you physically active after eating? (The combination of exercise and certain foods can spark a reaction.)

Make a list of the foods you suspect and go on to the next step.

ELIMINATION DIET

All you need to know to conquer food allergy can be stated in two words: expose, dispose. But be sure you've exposed the right foods before you dispose of them.

An elimination diet should always be done with a doctor's supervision. The basic premise is that you first clear your system by excluding from the diet: (1) potent allergens such as milk, wheat, eggs, corn, and nuts; (2) suspect allergens from your food diary list; (3) suspect allergens from skin or lab tests and medical history; and (4) vitamin pills and, if possible, medication.

Every allergist has his or her own way of administering the diet, and every diet should be custom-tailored to the patient's individual needs.

Let's assume a man we'll call Dan has multiple allergies. His elimination diet, at first, is Spartan. He subsists mainly on fresh meats, poultry, rice, noncitrus fruits, vegetables, and water. For the first few days he feels nervous and irritable due to "withdrawal" symptoms, but after a week he starts to improve. By the end of two weeks, Dan's system is cleared of allergens and to his delight, all his symptoms are gone.

Now begins the challenge—the gradual reintroduction of foods, one by one, at intervals of 3–7 days. A typical challenge starts with any fruits and vegetables that were eliminated, then proceeds to poultry, eggs, fish, red meat, and dairy products. Cocoa, sugars, nuts, and grains come last.

The long trial-and-error process isn't necessarily conclusive. If symptoms don't improve with an elimination diet, they're probably not related to allergy. Also, some foods have to be tested several times to confirm a cause-and-effect relationship.

When symptoms appear the first time a food is added and not the second, there could be several explanations:

- Dan isn't really allergic to the food. He was having a delayed reaction to some other food he ate earlier.

- Dan had a stressful day, a viral infection, or allergic reactions to other substances, which lowered his tolerance threshold.

- Dan can tolerate small amounts of the food. Corn-on-the-cob gives him symptoms, for instance, but a few kernels of corn in vegetable soup don't affect him.

- Dan ate the food in a different form. Cooking, baking, and mixing with other ingredients can change a food's chemistry.

You see how complicated this process is, and why you mustn't get frustrated. Total patience is essential!

OTHER TESTS

The streamlined version of the elimination diet may work if you suspect only one or two foods and your reactions are mild.

Say you choose wheat. For the next two weeks, avoid all forms of wheat, then see how you feel. If your symptoms diminish, you're probably on track. Reintroduce wheat for three consecutive meals, and watch yourself closely. If symptoms return, you may have your villain.

Some physicians claim to be able to identify food allergies by injecting small amounts of food extracts under the skin or squirting them under the tongue. Cutaneous and sublingual provocation tests, however, are unproven and experimental. So are two other food challenge tests: the kinetic muscle strength test and the pulse response. Kinesiology testing involves measuring muscle strength after food ingestion or sublingual application of food extracts. The pulse test, devised in the 1930s, measures pulse rate after eating certain foods. An increase is supposed to signal allergy. There is no evidence that either method has any value in identifying allergies.

THE BEST TEST

The DBPCFC—double-blind, placebo-controlled food challenge—is considered the "gold standard" for food allergies and the final answer when simpler diagnostic measures fail. It should never be used for patients with a history of anaphylaxis.

The DBPCFC works this way: Let's take our friend Dan, who by now has a fairly good idea what he's allergic to, but would like confirmation. Once again, he eats only simple, unprocessed, nonallergenic foods for two weeks. Then the doctor gives him a small opaque capsule of powdered food to swallow. At least Dan *thinks* it's powdered food, but it could be a placebo, an inert substance used as a control.

Ideally, neither Dan nor the doctor administering the test knows which capsule is food and which isn't. That way, there are no inadvertent psychological clues. A doctor, for instance, might be more alert when he's giving the actual allergen. If neither Dan nor the doctor knows what's in the capsules, Dan's reaction—or lack of it—will be based strictly on physiological factors.

The test is expensive, time-consuming, and not 100 percent reliable because of the difficulty in producing everyday foods in capsule form, but it has another important use. If the doctor suspected Dan's symptoms were *not* due to a food allergy, and could prove this to Dan, then they could start to look elsewhere for the real source of the problem.

Let's assume, however, that test results were conclusive. Dan exposed the foods to which he's allergic. Now he needs a diet that disposes of them.

CHAPTER 11

LIVING WITH
FOOD ALLERGY

You *can* live happily ever after, even with food allergies. If you like to spend time in the kitchen, many cookbooks offer recipes to accommodate specific needs—egg-free, milk-free, mold-free diets, whatever—and various combinations.

If you don't like to cook, that's fine, too, because the simplest, purest, freshest foods (fruits, vegetables, salads) are best for you. Go for recipes with the fewest ingredients, and leave the fancy sauces to the gourmets.

You may be one of the rare persons who reacts severely to a food. If so, NEVER eat it again. Your sensitivity will not diminish. A mild reaction is different. After you've abstained from the food for several months, your allergist may suggest you try a small amount. Here's the story of one patient.

A lifelong obesity-fighter, Susie M. hadn't had ice cream for several years when she discovered nonfat frozen yogurt. It was creamy, delicious, nutritious, and low-calorie. What a find!

A week into her frozen yogurt binge, however, she awoke one morning with a large canker sore on her tongue. She'd had canker sores before, though never quite so painful, and she assumed this would clear by itself as the others had done.

She made no connection with frozen yogurt. The soothing coolness seemed to help the soreness, in fact, and she increased her consumption. Finally, her tongue swelled to the point where she could neither talk nor eat.

The doctor prescribed antibiotics, which reduced the swelling, but it took months of eliminating and adding foods before Susie discovered the culprit was sugar. Like Francesca, she had brought on her allergy by overindulging.

The problem is still with Susie, although now she can tolerate one small dessert every three to four days. The irony is that cutting sweets from her diet has given her the beautiful slim figure she always wanted.

Food allergies can disappear for months, years, and sometimes the rest of your life. Once you return to a food you've been allergic to, your tolerance will be low. Start very gently, with small amounts every few days. Don't be lulled into thinking that because you can handle a little, you can handle a lot more. Your sensitivity can come back worse than before—and with a whole new set of symptoms.

Moderation is the rule even when you think you're "cured." Don't tempt trouble by eating too much of a good thing.

LABELS

Shopping for food with your new knowledge will take longer, and you may have to go to several stores to get the products you want, but your time will be well spent and can save you from suffering later.

Be vigilant in checking labels. Read the list each time you buy a product; ingredients can change. If the food or additive you're allergic to is not listed, look again. Foods often masquerade under different names. For example:

- *Sugar:* a.k.a. sucrose, glucose, lactose, maltose, dextrose, fructose, corn sweetener, maltodextrin, honey, corn syrup, maple syrup, rice syrup, malt syrup, molasses, fruit concentrate.

- *Milk:* casein, caseinate, sodium caseinate, whey, lactose, lactoglobulin, lactalbumen, curds.

- *Egg:* albumin, yolk, vitellin, ovovitellin, livetin, globulin, ovomucin, ovomucoid.

- *Wheat:* gluten, graham flour, monosodium glutamate (MSG), hydrolyzed vegetable protein (HVP), durum flour, semolina, bulgur.

Be skeptical of all claims on labels. The words "pure," "natural," and "healthy" are meaningless. "No preservatives added" often means that preservatives are already in one or more ingredients. "String beans" doesn't mention what pesticides or fungicides were used to grow the vegetables, or what chemicals were used to process them.

Cool Whip and Coffee-mate, hailed as "nondairy" products, contain caseinate, a milk derivative. Sweet'n Low "sugar substitute" contains "nutritive dextrose"—but you need a magnifying glass to find it listed on the packet. Manufacturers often sneak a bit of wheat into rice, rye, and potato breads—not enough to matter unless you happen to be allergic to wheat. Suspect all baked goods that rise.

Also, many allergy-producing foods show up in unexpected places; soy and casein (milk) in canned tuna, corn fillers in vitamin and mineral pills, corn in chewing gum and instant tea, benzoate in soy sauce, wheat in pea soup and vodka, egg in marshmallows, milk in hot dogs, fish oils in envelope and postage stamp glue.

Be especially wary of unlabeled bakery goods, fast-food and restaurant fare, and dining at parties and friends' homes. Allergens often lurk where least expected. For more information on labels and new food products, call the Food Allergy Network (FAN) at 800-929-4040.

MILK-FREE DIET

You'll probably find yourself eating more meals at home, or at least preparing your own lunches instead of flirting with fate in the office cafeteria.

If milk is your problem, your symptoms are likely to be digestive: bloating, abdominal cramps, flatulence, diarrhea, constipation. Headaches, earaches, rhinitis, eczema, and asthma are also associated with cow's milk.

Soy milk is a popular alternative, and has a slightly stronger flavor that benefits from chilling. It's another potent allergen, however, and should be used with restraint. Milk and soy allergies are particularly common in infants and children.

Other possibilities are goat's milk, nut milks, coconut milk, fruit juice, and tea. Kosher products labeled "parve" or "pareve" don't contain milk. People with lactase deficiency can usually eat yogurt, which contains its own lactase. Be sure the label specifies "live cultures." Pasteurization destroys the enzyme.

Depending on your degree of sensitivity, you may be able to tolerate the small amounts of milk in bread and some other baked goods. Milk is fairly easy to avoid because it's found where you most expect it, in dairy products such as butter, cheese, cottage cheese, and ice cream. But it also turns up in such less-obvious places as:

- Cakes and cake mixes, doughnuts, fritters, cookies

- Carob

- Chocolate candies, nougat

- Cream sauces, gravies

- Cream soups, chowders, bisques

- Custards, puddings, soufflés

- Margarine

- Mashed potatoes

- Meat loaf, sausage, luncheon meats, hot dogs, milk-fed veal

- Noodles (macaroni, spaghetti)

- Pancakes, waffles

- Potato chips (some)

- Salad dressings (some)
- Sherbets

HINT: Be a compulsive label reader. The effort will pay off.

WHEAT-FREE DIET

Allergy to wheat tends to blossom in the spring, when related grasses are filling the air with pollen and lowering tolerance thresholds. Like milk, wheat tends to cause gastric distress, eczema, and hay fever, as well as asthma and more serious reactions.

Substitutes for wheat include corn, potato, barley, oat, soy, and rice flours, sago and arrowroot starches. Well-sifted combinations tend to be more palatable than single flours. An easy replacement for a cup of wheat flour is ½ cup of rye flour and ½ cup of potato flour.

Wheat is prevalent in so many products that avoiding it is something of a challenge. Along with the usual cereals, pasta, and bakery goods, suspect wheat in:

- Alcoholic beverages, including ale, beer, gin, and some wines
- Anything breaded or deep-fried
- Baked beans
- Candies
- Cheese spreads
- Chili
- Fruit (stewed, thickened)
- Meat loaf, sausages
- Meats, canned and processed
- Monosodium glutamate (MSG)

- Pancakes, waffles
- Postum
- Potato chips (some)
- Salad dressings (some)
- Soufflés, custards, puddings, most desserts
- Soups
- Vitamins, especially vitamin E
- White sauce, gravies

HINT: Steer clear of unlabeled products, bakeries, and Italian restaurants.

EGG-FREE DIET

Allergy to egg, especially the white, is more common in children than adults. Reactions to a tiny amount can be instantaneous and severe.

Milder reactions generally target the skin and respiratory and gastrointestinal tracts. Sensitivity tends to be long-lasting, so don't break out the omelette pan too soon.

Egg substitutes that do not contain egg whites are useful in recipes. Or you can replace one egg with a mixture of 1 teaspoon egg-free baking powder, 1½ tablespoons oil, and ½ tablespoons water.

These products often (not always) contain egg:

- Anything French-fried or batter-fried
- Baking powder
- Bread, baked goods
- Candies, marshmallows
- Cookies (especially macaroons, chocolate chip)
- Creamed foods and sauces; tartar sauce

- Crêpes
- Custards, puddings, soufflés, zabayon, whipped desserts, floating island, meringue
- Deviled or coddled foods
- Frostings
- Lecithin
- Mayonnaise
- Mixed salads (tuna, chicken, potato)
- Noodles (macaroni, spaghetti)
- Pies (pumpkin, lemon, custard, banana)
- Root beer (egg is used to produce foam)
- Timbales
- Waffles
- Wines (some)

HINT: Watch out for shiny baked goods with an egg white glaze.

SUGAR-FREE DIET

Sugar is usually eaten in a form so refined that its allergenic qualities have been lost in the manufacturing process. Nevertheless, sugar allergies exist.

Some people who cannot tolerate cane sugar can eat other forms: grape, corn, rice, and maple syrups, honey, molasses, and beet sugar.

Susie, the patient mentioned at the beginning of this chapter, was not so lucky. Once sensitized, she found she could not tolerate any kind of sugar, not even the fructose in fruits. Along with canker sores and mouth swelling, she would have cramps, bloating, and diarrhea.

Sorbitol, xylitol, and mannitol were too closely related to sugar for Susie to use, and even the maltodextrin in powdered

NutraSweet provoked symptoms. The only sweeteners she could handle were saccharin, which in very high doses causes cancer in mice, and pure aspartame, which does not contain maltodextrin. She now buys special products, such as Dannon Non-Fat Vanilla Yogurt sweetened only with aspartame, and has shifted her sweet tooth to her favorite unsweet foods—bean soups, (homemade) tuna sandwiches, stewed chicken, nonfat potato chips, and so on.

You may be surprised to learn there's sugar in some brands of the following:

- Beer, wine, gin, rum
- Breads, muffins, rolls
- Caramel coloring
- Cheese spreads
- Chicken soup and most canned soups
- Chinese food
- Crêpes, pancakes, waffles
- Mixed nuts
- Peanut butter
- Salad dressings, catsup, tomato sauce
- Sugar substitutes
- Sugar-free foods (honey, corn syrup, and maltodextrin are still sugars)
- Vitamin pills and supplements

HINT: If a product's ingredients aren't listed, don't buy it.

NUT-FREE DIET

Reaction to nuts can be swift and lethal. They're one of the foods most closely associated with anaphylaxis. In milder cases, nuts can cause skin rashes and gastric distress.

Peanuts, strictly speaking, are a legume related to peas, and not a member of the nut family. They're such a potent allergen, however, and so commonly thought to be a nut, they're included here.

Excluding such obvious sources as almond paste, nut oils, and nut butters, foods that usually contain nuts are:

- Cakes, cookies, all bakery desserts
- Candies, granola, high-energy bars
- Cereals
- Chinese, Korean, Thai restaurant foods
- Grain breads
- Ice creams, frozen desserts
- Salad dressings

HINT: Keep your eyes open. The world is full of nuts.

CORN-FREE DIET

One of the sneakiest of foods, corn can creep into almost every meal in one form or another. The corn-allergic person can be so sensitive that he or she can't lick a stamp because of corn in the glue, or drink milk because of minute traces of cornstarch from the paper container.

Eczema and abdominal and respiratory problems are associated with this allergy.

Corn-free diets are relatively easy to prepare because few recipes call for corn products. Various starches such as potato, arrowroot, taro, and tapioca can substitute as thickeners, and corn-free baking powder is available in health food stores.

Corn shows up in so many unlikely places, sensitive persons must be diligent in reading labels. Avoid not only the word "corn," but all sugars ending in "ose," which are corn derivatives. Some unexpected sources might be:

- Ale, beer, gin, whiskey

- Aspartame (NutraSweet)
- Aspirin, cough medicine
- Bakery goods
- Baking powder
- Candies
- Carbonated drinks
- Catsup
- Coffee (instant)
- Fruits (canned, frozen)
- Gravies, soups
- Ham, bacon, sausage, hot dogs, lunch meats
- Ice cream, sherbet
- Jams, jellies
- Margarine
- Peanut butter
- Plastic food wrap
- Salad dressings
- Sorbitol, mannitol
- Table salt
- Tamales, tortillas, enchiladas
- Toothpaste

HINT: Stay out of Mexican restaurants.

ASPIRIN (SALICYLATE)-FREE DIET

Aspirin—acetylsalicylic acid—is great for soothing headaches, but sometimes it can be a pain in itself. Certain unlucky people find that aspirin provokes hives, gastric distress, a runny nose, swollen eyes, asthma, or worse. These folks should not only avoid aspirin but all related compounds: anti-inflammatory drugs such as naproxen and ibuprofen, as well as foods and drugs that contain tartrazine (yellow food dye no. 5) or sodium benzoate, a preservative.

For pain relief, acetaminophen (Tylenol, Datril) can usually be substituted safely.

Foods not allowed on a salicylate-free diet include:

- All alcoholic beverages except gin and scotch
- Almonds, Brazil nuts
- Apples, apricots, berries, cherries, grapes, nectarines, oranges, peaches, pears, melons
- Bakery goods
- Candies, gum
- Canned vegetables
- Cheese (processed)
- Cucumbers, peppers, olives, radishes, tomato sauce
- Dried fruits, including raisins and prunes
- Flavorings: mint, cloves, curry
- Hot dogs, lunch meats
- Ice cream, Jell-O
- Jams, jellies, honey
- Margarine
- Soft drinks, mineral water
- Sweetened breads
- Wine, wine vinegar

HINT: Beware of all foods artificially colored or flavored.

MOLD-FREE DIET

Molds can be avoided effectively, but not entirely. Many are harmless; others can be dangerous. Some molds enhance the flavor of foods, especially cheeses. Blue cheese owes its distinctive taste to *Penicillium roqueforti*; Camembert is ripened by *Penicillium camemberti*. If you're allergic to penicillin, be wary of these cheeses.

Molds are also useful in food processing. They produce amylase, an enzyme used to make breads, and play a strong role in the production of fermented products, from soy sauce and sake to sugar-cured hams.

If you're mold-sensitive, consider a few suggestions:

1. Don't smell foods to see if they're spoiled. Inhaling the spores can set off a reaction.

2. Discard all fresh foods that appear discolored, shriveled, or show signs of mold. Spit out anything, especially a nut, that tastes bitter.

3. Discard any of the following foods that show signs of mold: soft cheeses, sour cream, yogurt, bakery goods, flour, whole grains, corn and corn products, nuts and nut butters, dried peas and beans.

4. You needn't discard hard cheeses, hard fruits, and hard vegetables (such as carrots, celery, or cabbage). Cut away the moldy spot and a cubic inch around it.

5. With jams and jellies, spoon off the surface mold, then use a clean spoon to scoop out the area around it. If mold goes deeper, discard the jam.

6. Don't let mold-contaminated utensils touch any other food or cooking surface. Wash all utensils and cutting boards with hot soapy water.

Flu-like symptoms are often the first indication of mold allergy. Headaches, gastric upset, joint pain, and muscle soreness may occur hours to days after exposure.

Yeast, one of the most widely occurring molds in foods, has no replacement as a leavening agent (causing baked goods to rise). Toasted 100 percent rye bread, cut horizontally into thin, crusty slices, helps make a passable sandwich. Fresh lemon juice can season salads instead of vinegar, but skip dried spices. They're loaded with molds.

If you're sensitive to any form of fungi, shop often, buy small amounts of fresh food, check date labels on packages and cartons, and don't leave leftovers sitting around the kitchen. Last night's dinner, refrigerated, is good for only 24 hours. Let your guests take home the chocolate cake. Molds thrive on the sugar in your body.

Some foods to exclude or use sparingly:

- Bakery goods made with yeast, or any "day old" bakery goods

- Cheese (all types including cottage cheese)

- Chocolate

- Deep-fried foods (bread crumb batter)

- Fermented drinks (beer, brandy, gin, ginger ale, root beer, rum, whiskey, wine, vodka)

- Foods containing citric acid

- Fruit (dried, candied, overripe)

- Fruit juices (all types except fresh-squeezed)

- Hamburger (unless fresh-frozen or freshly ground)

- Malt products (candy, cereals, malted milk)

- Melons, especially cantaloupe

- Multi-B vitamins

- Mushrooms, truffles

- Peanuts

- Pickles, pickled meats (pastrami, tongue), pickled vegetables, green olives, sauerkraut

- Smoked fish and meats

- Sour cream, buttermilk

- Soy sauce, tofu (soy curd)

- Teas

- Tomato products (usually made from overripe tomatoes)
- Vinegar, vinegar-containing foods (mayonnaise, catsup, mustard)

HINT: When in doubt, throw it out.

SULFITES

Sulfites are chemicals added to many foods to preserve color and the appearance of freshness. Until fairly recently, sulfites (including sodium and potassium bisulfite or metabisulfite, sulfur dioxide, and sodium sulfite) were used extensively on fruits and vegetables in salad bars, delis, and restaurants.

Because sulfites caused breathing difficulties in some people, and others suffered fatal allergic reactions, the FDA issued a regulation requiring food establishments to list sulfiting agents on their menus. Until we have "sulfite police" to look over the shoulders of chefs and caterers, however, you'd best beware of all foods you see in deli cases, salad bars, buffet spreads, and generally "on display." Don't take the word of waiters or waitresses who may not know what's going on in the kitchen.

Many sulfites are added in the manufacturing process, so whenever you buy packaged or prepared foods, read the labels. Be especially careful of:

- Anything dried, especially shellfish and fruit
- Bread and cake mixes (some)
- Cakes and pastries containing dried fruit
- Commercial bread
- Grapes, mainly from California
- Guacamole (unless homemade)
- Nut products (some)
- Potatoes (instant or dehydrated), potato salad

- Vegetables (dehydrated for use in salads, soups, seasonings, dressings, and food mixes)
- Wines (some), soft drinks, beer

HINT: When in doubt, don't eat out.

MIGRAINES

Migraine headaches vary in intensity from mild to disabling. They're usually pounding, one-sided, and accompanied by nausea. Classic migraine attacks are preceded by auras—strange sensations of sounds, smells, and/or visual distortions. Common migraines are more prevalent, milder, and have no aura, but may occur more frequently.

More common in women than men, migraines are associated with both food allergies and intolerances. They can also be triggered by physical agents such as sunlight, heat and cold, and by stress, fatigue, or a viral infection.

Foods, however, are fairly easy to control. Avoid prolonged fasting, skipping meals, or eating large amounts of carbohydrates at one sitting.

Migraine-sufferers are often sensitive to one or more of these substances:

- *Caffeine*—found in coffee, colas, some headache pills.
- *Ethanol*—found in alcoholic beverages. Beer, champagne, and red wine are particular offenders.
- *Nitrites, MSG, sulfites, tartrazine*—found in processed foods, beverages, medication.
- *Phenylethylamine*—found in chocolate.
- *Tyramine*—found in aged or sharp cheese, anchovies, avocados, bacon, bananas, broad beans, canned figs, caviar, chicken liver, ham, hot dogs, luncheon meats, pickled herring, yogurt.

Other possible migraine triggers are: aspartame, beef, cane sugar, citrus fruits (mainly oranges,) corn, eggs, deep-fried foods, milk, nuts, onions, peanuts, pork, products containing yeast, raisins, seafood, tea, wheat.

These foods are *not* likely to cause migraines:

* Cottage cheese and cream cheese

* Desserts sweetened with other than cane sugar

* Fruit: apples, apricots, berries, cherries, grapes, peaches, pears

* Meat: chicken, duck, lamb, turkey, veal

* Vegetables: artichokes, asparagus, beets, broccoli, carrots, cauliflower, celery, cucumber, eggplant, green beans, lettuce, parsnips, peas, potatoes, sprouts.

HINT: The three Cs—coffee, cheese, and chocolate—are the main migraine suspects.

ROTARY DIET

The first rotary diet, developed in the 1930s by pioneer allergist Herbert J. Rinkel, M.D., was based on a simple principle: It usually takes four days for a food to "clear" the body. When a food is eaten and not repeated for four days, the body has time to get rid of the troublemaking antibodies. They cannot accumulate, and the patient avoids getting symptoms.

Take Tony P., a pasta-loving Italian who developed a sensitivity to tomatoes. He stopped eating all tomato products for three months, and his dermatitis cleared up dramatically. After a few weeks of experimenting, he found he could eat a single helping of spaghetti Bolognese every four days and not break out in a rash. By rotating his foods and diversifying his diet, he could occasionally enjoy "forbidden fruit."

Rotation makes sense for many reasons. It helps you identify food allergens, lets you eat small portions of the foods you're allergic to, and keeps you from developing allergies to new foods due to overexposure.

You'll probably want to fine-tune the diet to your personal needs. Here's how to start:

1. Take a week or two to clear your body of allergens by excluding all the foods that seem to give you symptoms.

2. Build a new diet around primary foods: fish, meat, poultry, fruits, vegetables, grains, and dairy products, as close to their natural state as possible. Avoid packaged or processed foods.

3. Select a minimum number of foods for each meal, and fill up on large portions, rather than eating small portions of various foods.

4. Don't eat the same food more than once a day even if you're not allergic to it. Some doctors will tell you not to eat foods in the same botanical family more than once a day, but other doctors believe that cross-reactivity—reacting to all foods in the same family—is rare. You'll have to experiment. (Food families are listed in Appendix E.)

5. Don't forget to rotate beverages, seasonings, cooking oils, and any additives and preservatives you can't avoid.

6. Be sure to distinguish between foods in the same family and foods containing the same ingredient. Oranges and lemons, for example, are in the same food family, but in most cases, you can drink orange juice at breakfast and lemonade at dinner. Orange juice and rainbow sherbet, on the other hand, both *contain* oranges, so the four-day rule would apply.

7. Keeping a notebook will help you remember what you ate and when. You'll find yourself experimenting with various foods and reaching a point where you know exactly how often you can eat a particular food without reacting.

Beth B., a schoolteacher who had excluded corn from her diet for years, began to rotate her foods, and found she could tolerate one corn product a day. Two corn products, however, exceeded her threshold and started her sneezing. You may find you can rotate certain foods on a one-, two-, or three-day basis.

Even if all you do is diversify your diet and limit your intake of various foods, this is a wise regime. The rotary diet has lasted for many years because it works. A great number of books on the subject are available to provide tips, recipes, and substitutions.

Try it. It's easier than you think.

PART IV

ASTHMA

Over 12 million Americans suffer from asthma, also called reactive lung disease. It is a chronic ailment that's continually on the rise. The increase most likely stems from the proliferation in modern life of such triggers as allergens, air pollution, and stress factors.

An asthma attack occurs when the airways (bronchial tubes) contract, become swollen and inflamed, and produce excess mucus, blocking the passage of air. The result is that breathing becomes exceedingly difficult. The patient experiences one or more of these symptoms: dry cough, wheezing, shortness of breath, chest tightness, and coughing up sputum.

After repeated episodes, lung tissue loses elasticity, causing a gradual decline in function. Fatigue often sets in from the extra effort to take in air. Symptoms may get worse at night.

The severity of an attack can vary greatly, from mild to life-threatening. Reactions can also be minor on one occasion and major on another.

There are three types of asthma:

Acute asthma is a sudden attack that requires immediate attention. It can last minutes or days. When it's severe, it's a life-threatening emergency. Distress symptoms include:

- Intense coughing, wheezing, shortness of breath.

- Breathing that's shallow and fast or very slow.
- Cyanosis—a gray or bluish tint to the skin, particularly around the mouth.
- Difficulty concentrating or talking.
- Hunched shoulders.
- Inability to walk or move without gasping for breath.
- Nostrils that flare with breathing.
- Tightness in the chest.
- Peak flow numbers below 50 percent (see pages 114–116).

Chronic asthma produces continual symptoms of varying degrees and is caused by ongoing airway inflammation.

Nocturnal asthma is very common and may have to do with the body's "internal clocks" or circadian cycles. Due to these natural body rhythms, lungs function best around four in the afternoon and worst around four in the morning.

Night asthma problems can also be due to decreased levels of body chemicals that open the airways, a drop in body temperature that constricts the airways, or a delayed allergic reaction that acts as a trigger.

All types of asthma can be prevented, monitored, and controlled with medication.

CHAPTER 12

NEW APPROACHES

All that wheezes is not asthma. Doctors now know that a number of other medical conditions—vocal cord abnormalities, airway obstruction from foreign bodies or tumors, lung and heart diseases—can cause symptoms that mimic asthma. For this reason, several highly accurate diagnostic tests have been developed, some within the last few years.

Medication has changed, too. Improved beta-agonist drugs (Proventil, Alupent) have specific action on the airways and fewer side effects than their predecessors (Bronkosol, Primatene Mist).

Recent research has indicated that inflammation of the lining of the airways is at the root of asthma attacks. This finding has led doctors, more and more, to reverse previous thinking that asthma was the result of constricted bronchial muscles. Today, many physicians start therapy by treating inflammation and irritation and prescribing corticosteroids (CCS) as first-line medication for anyone with moderate to severe asthma (more than two episodes a week). Then they add bronchodilators, drugs to relax and open the airways.

All steroids have side effects, however, and the National Jewish Center for Immunology and Respiratory Medicine in Denver, Colorado, has a major program directed at finding therapies to replace them.

As you read this, scientists across the country are seeking a better understanding of asthma. Their main goal is prevention—the elimination of asthmatic episodes by careful monitoring, and the use of medication to hold down inflammation.

Research centered on physiological and emotional aspects of the disease will also lead to improved treatments with emphasis on self-management.

TRIGGERS

If you have asthma, your airways are almost always inflamed, and therefore more sensitive to various triggers. The ones most likely to set off an asthma attack are:

ALLERGENS—Eighty percent of asthmatics have positive skin tests to such airborne substances as dust, pollen, molds, cockroach particles, and dander from furry or feathery animals. This type of allergic asthma is most common in children over 3 and adults under 50.

IRRITANTS—The long list includes aerosol sprays, strong odors, industrial and occupational chemicals, car exhaust, indoor and outdoor air pollution, cigarette smoke, and smoke from wood-burning or kerosene stoves and fireplaces.

MEDICAL CONDITIONS—Gastroesophageal reflux or GER (leaks of stomach acid into the esophagus, especially at night) is a common trigger.

MEDICATION—Be cautious with aspirin and other nonsteroidal anti-inflammatory agents such as ibuprofen and naproxen, and avoid beta-blockers. (Don't confuse beta-blockers, or beta-adrenergic-blocking drugs, which are used to treat migraine, heart disease, high blood pressure, and glaucoma, with beta-agonists or beta-adrenergic drugs, which are used to treat asthma.)

EXERCISE—Strenuous exertion causes a narrowing of the airways, or bronchospasm, in about 80 percent of people with asthma. (See Chapter 14.)

STRESS, ANXIETY, ANGER—Emotional upsets can bring on symptoms, but asthma starts in the lungs, not the head.

FOODS AND FOOD ADDITIVES—Avoid products with tartrazine (yellow dye no. 5) and sulfites. In the digestive process, sulfites mix with stomach acids and become sulfuric acid, a gas. The gas travels up through the esophagus, is breathed in, and provokes symptoms.

COLDS, INFLUENZA, BRONCHITIS, AND OTHER VIRAL RESPIRATORY INFECTIONS—Wash your hands frequently during flu season or when someone in the household is sick. If your doctor approves, get an annual flu shot.

SINUSITIS—Inflamed mucous membranes lining the sinus cavities may cause nocturnal symptoms.

WEATHER—Extremes of temperature, windy conditions, changes in humidity or barometric pressure affect everyone differently. Chilly weather may trigger asthma for persons sensitive to cold, yet be beneficial to those with pollen allergy.

HORMONAL CHANGES IN WOMEN—Premenstrual hormone changes and pregnancy can heighten susceptibility.

MECHANICAL RESPONSES—Sneezing, coughing, laughing, yelling, hyperventilation (deep, rapid, "heavy" breathing) can lead to wheezing. Some people with asthma have to take medication before making love.

EARLY WARNINGS

There are two ways to monitor yourself to prevent or lessen the severity of an impending attack. One is to become familiar with the physical signals that precede an episode, so that you're alerted in time to take steps. These signals are unique to each person and are usually (but not always) the same for each episode.

Some of the most common early warning signs are:

- Allergic shiners (dark circles under eyes)
- Changes in breathing
- Change in the color, amount, or thickness of mucus
- Coughing
- Dry mouth
- Feeling tired, touchy, sad, or depressed
- Hay fever—runny, stuffy nose, sneezing
- Headache
- Increased sensory awareness
- Inability to sleep
- Itchy throat or chin
- Rapid heartbeat
- Vague heaviness and tightness in chest

PEAK FLOW METERS

A more scientific way to monitor yourself is with a hand-held plastic device called a peak flow meter. It's a small cylinder with numbers along the shaft, and its purpose is to measure the peak expiratory flow rate (PEFR)—how fast and hard you can blow air out of your lungs.

The peak flow meter is small and easy to carry and can be used at work, home, school, or wherever you go. A four-year-old child can be taught to master it.

The device tells how well your lungs are working and the degree of airway blockage. It not only warns of possible breathing difficulties but also helps you and your physician determine which medications are best for you, how much to take, how often, when to stop taking them, and when to seek emergency care. In most cases, medication can correct the problem fairly quickly and restore your peak flow to normal.

With your doctor's help, you can determine your normal airflow, depending on your age, weight, height, and sex. This is called your "personal best" or "peak capacity," and is the highest number you usually obtain over a two-week period when your asthma is controlled.

You'll also know what to do when the value drops, indicating that you're entering the danger zone and need to ward off an attack. Learn to recognize all three zones:

GREEN ZONE—A reading at 80–100 percent of personal best signals all clear.

YELLOW ZONE—A reading at 50–80 percent of peak capacity signals caution. It may mean the beginning of an episode and a warning for you to rest, do breathing exercises (see Chapter 14), take medication, and avoid triggers until you get back into the green zone.

RED ZONE—A reading below 50 percent signals danger! Take rescue medicine (prearranged with your doctor) and seek immediate medical help.

Using the meter at least two (preferably three times) a day will provide a picture of how your lungs are working and help you recognize the physical sensations that precede trouble. Your doctor will probably ask you to keep a daily diary of peak flow readings, to record which drugs you take and in what amounts, and to bring the diary with you to your medical appointments.

For best results with your peak flow meter:

- Set the scale to zero.

- Take the reading in the same position every time, preferably standing up. If you can't stand up, choose a comfortable sitting or reclining position.

- Breathe in deeply.

- Close your lips around the mouthpiece.

- Don't let your tongue block the mouth of the meter. Try not to cough.

- Blow out as hard and fast as you can without bending over.

- Write down the value you see on the scale.

- Take two more readings and record the highest of the three in your peak flow diary.

Peak flow meters sell for around $20 to $40, don't require a prescription, and are as vital to the asthmatic as blood-pressure kits are to the hypertense. Most health insurance covers peak flow meters. You can call the Allergy and Asthma Network (see Appendix A) to order one at reduced cost.

CHOOSING A DOCTOR

When your primary-care physician recommends an asthma specialist, it will either be an allergist or a pulmonologist (lung specialist). Not all allergists and pulmonologists specialize in asthma, however, so check this out in advance.

The first thing the specialist will do is take a detailed history of your allergic and asthmatic background. Be prepared to supply times, dates, and places attacks occurred, along with known and suspected triggers, whether sleep was interrupted, how many work or school days you missed, all previous treatment, including medication, and its efficacy.

Prevention magazine suggests taking the advice of Dr. Tom

Plaut, author and nationally recognized expert in the treatment of asthma. According to Dr. Plaut, you should look for a doctor who:

1. Provides detailed written instructions and preprinted forms that he or she individualizes for you
2. Shows you how to use a peak flow meter
3. Shows you how to use an inhaler
4. Works with you as a partner to control your asthma.

If your asthma doesn't improve significantly after three months, look for another doctor.

DIAGNOSIS

When your medical history and physical exam point to asthma, your doctor may recommend one or more of the following diagnostic aids:

ARTERIAL GAS TESTS—to determine oxygen and carbon dioxide levels in blood. Greater or lesser amounts can be signals of breathing problems.

BLOOD TESTS—to check blood sugar level, which may indicate diabetes (which interferes with the effectiveness of asthma medication), or to ascertain the presence of large numbers of eosinophils, a kind of white blood cell, which indicates the asthma is related to allergy. RAST, PRIST, and ELISA tests (see Chapter 5) are also used to measure IgE levels and responses to specific allergens.

CHEST X RAY—usually normal in an asthmatic; should only be used to rule out heart disease, cystic fibrosis, bronchitis, pneumonia and other lung diseases, or when complications such as rib fractures are suspected.

PULMONARY FUNCTION TESTS—to check lung capability. Spirometry requires a technician and a special device that records on a graph the amount of air you're exhaling. Asthmatics have a hard time blowing out air and take longer to exhale. The spirometer also measures the degree of airway obstruction and the effects of medication. If lung capacity doesn't improve with bronchodilation, other problems such as emphysema may be present.

Self-administered peak flow tests, properly performed, are equally reliable lung function monitors.

SINUS X RAY—to determine presence of postnasal drip and/or sinusitis, a common asthma trigger.

SKIN TESTING—to evaluate the effects of airborne irritants and confirm that wheezing is allergic asthma rather than lung disease. (A blood test for specific IgE can do the same.)

SPUTUM ANALYSIS—for eosinophils, molds, and/or mucus plugs that obstruct the air passages.

The doctor may also recommend an oral challenge (oral bronchial provocation) test to confirm sensitivity to foods, drugs (particularly aspirin), and additives (mainly sulfites). You swallow tiny doses of the suspected substance at intervals of 10–20 minutes, and the doctor monitors forced exhalation.

In an inhalation challenge test, the allergens are breathed in, not swallowed, and in an exercise challenge test, you work out on a treadmill, rowing machine, or exercise bicycle. All challenges produce symptoms and must be closely supervised. The main usefulness of these tests is in discovering which medications are most effective in stopping the response.

CHAPTER 13

MODERN MEDICATION

Once asthma has been determined and other possible diagnoses ruled out, you and your doctor should work together to develop a treatment program that uses the least amount of medication with the fewest side effects. There is no set formula for treating asthma. Each person must experiment to find the drug or combination of drugs that works best.

Most asthma medications fall into two groups: anti-inflammatory drugs, to reduce redness and swelling, and bronchodilators, to open the airways or keep them open.

ANTI-INFLAMMATORY DRUGS

These medications are the new focus of asthma therapy because they treat the underlying inflammation that causes airway obstruction. The most effective anti-inflammatory medications are corticosteroids (CCS) and cromolyn sodium. CCS is frequently used in conjunction with bronchodilators for patients who require somewhat heavier medication, or for any asthmatic who wheezes more than two days a week.

Inhaled Steroids

Inhaled steroids, also called topical steroids—usually triamcinolone (Azmacort), flunisolide (AeroBid), or beclomethasone (Beclovent, Vanceril)—are not the same as the anabolic steroids used illegally by athletes. Inhaled CCS does not promote muscle growth, affect the liver, or cause sterility. It acts at the site of the disease and is absorbed into the lung tissue. Very little medication escapes to the bloodstream. Patients report better results with frequent use of lower doses than with occasional use of stronger doses.

Side effects are relatively minor for short-term usage, although some patients report hoarseness and coughing. Rinsing of the mouth after use is always advised to reduce the possibility of getting thrush, a yeast infection.

Ginny G., a longtime sufferer, had her first asthma attack in grammar school. She recalled playing basketball at recess and puffing and wheezing so badly that the school nurse phoned her mother to come pick her up. After that, Ginny was instructed to sit quietly on the bench while her classmates ran, jumped, and played.

Asthma followed Ginny to adulthood, and by the time she was 30 she was resigned to becoming an invalid—unable to run a few steps or climb stairs without wheezing, and forced to carry portable oxygen.

Oral steroids came to her rescue, especially in the cold of winter when her symptoms were at their worst. Side effects of the medication, however, made her moon-faced, overweight, and depressed.

All that changed when Ginny's new allergist prescribed inhaled steroids. She began to take six to eight puffs of beclomethasone daily. The new dosage was about 1 milligram, or one-fortieth of the 40-milligram pill she'd been swallowing. Amazingly, her attacks responded just as well to the weaker dosage.

The doctor explained what was happening: "Inhaled steroids go directly to your lungs. It's like shooting a pistol at a bull's-eye instead of spraying a volley of bullets into the air and hoping one will hit the target."

With her lowered dosage and successful treatment, Ginny's swelling subsided, her appetite returned to normal, and her mood was once again upbeat.

Doctors are optimistic about a newly available inhaled steroid. Budesonide, said to relieve croup, a viral infection that causes hoarseness and breathing difficulties in children, is also used to control nasal symptoms associated with allergies. Because the drug is potent, a smaller amount is needed, and patients are less likely to develop side effects.

Oral Steroids

Severe asthma that does not respond to the combination of bronchodilators and inhaled steroids sometimes requires stronger medicine. Oral steroids in tablet form—most commonly prednisone (Medicorten, Deltasone), prednisolone (Deltacortef), methylprednisolone (Medrol), and dexamethasone (Decadron)—are highly effective at reducing airway inflammation, decreasing mucus production, and enhancing the effects of bronchodilators.

Oral steroids can be used for short-term bursts or, in rare cases, for long-term treatment. They should always be taken with other asthma medication, never alone, and they have side effects even from minimal use. Less than 7.5 milligrams of prednisone daily may evoke stomach upset, mood changes, and weight gain. Fortunately, these are not devastating problems and do not preclude the use of oral CCS when required. After the medication stops, the symptoms disappear.

Extended use of oral steroids may give rise to more serious problems such as high blood pressure, fluid retention, easy bruisability, hair growth, muscle weakness, cataract formation, fragile bones, acne, and poor resistance to infection. Susceptible persons can develop diabetes and heart disease. Long-term use inhibits growth in children. Both children and adults should discontinue usage slowly.

Not everyone who takes steroids will get serious reactions. Nevertheless, oral steroids should only be used when absolutely necessary, and under the continued close supervision of a specialist. You can lessen risks by starting with the weakest possible dosage, adopting an alternate day regimen, and taking the pills in the morning, with breakfast.

Cromolyn

Cromolyn sodium, which has anti-inflammatory properties, acts best as a preventive, especially when asthma is induced by exercise, food and airborne allergens, or cold air. Patients whose asthma is triggered by other factors respond positively to cromolyn about 50 percent of the time, so it warrants a trial in most cases. Children have a slightly higher rate of success.

Cromolyn therapy is slow to work and may require four to eight weeks before you notice improvement. A single dose taken 5–60 minutes prior to contact with a trigger, however, can sometimes prevent symptoms for three or four hours.

One allergist gives severely asthmatic patients a month of the bronchodilator albuterol to open the windpipe and a week of oral steroids to reduce inflammation before starting preventive therapy with cromolyn. He also recommends using an inhaled bronchodilator along with cromolyn for the first month, to be sure the cromolyn reaches the lungs.

Inhaled cromolyn (Intal, Nasalcrom) is available in several inhalant devices (see Chapter 14). Side effects are negligible, in most cases limited to coughing and throat irritation. You can avoid this by sipping water after inhalation. Cromolyn is not recommended for pregnant women.

Nedocromil, a related product available elsewhere in the world, has just been approved for use in the United States. It appears to be as effective as cromolyn in reducing inflammation, and can be tried on asthmatics who have not responded to cromolyn.

BRONCHODILATORS

There are three types of bronchodilators: beta-agonists, methyl-xanthines, and anticholinergics.

Beta-agonists

These drugs, also called beta-adrenergic agents, work by relaxing the bronchial muscles to prevent their narrowing and to open the airways.

Best and newest of the beta-agonist drugs are albuterol (Proventil, Ventolin), bitolterol (Tornalate), pirbuterol (Maxair), and salmeterol (Serevent). They can be taken orally as pills or, more commonly, sprayed and inhaled.

When used in moderation, they're not habit-forming and have no long-term side effects. Short-term use, however, can provoke rapid heartbeat, dizziness, nervousness, nausea, and tremors. In case of chest pain, severe headache, delusions, or vomiting, call your doctor right away.

Methylxanthines

The second type of bronchodilator, methylxanthines, includes caffeine, theobromine, and the much-maligned theophylline, sold in tablet, capsule, or liquid form under more than fifty brand names, including Constant-T, Neulin, Slo-bid, Slo-Phyllin, Theo-24, Theo-Dur, Theolair, and Uniphyl.

From 1970 to 1990, theophylline was the prime drug in asthma treatment, but questions about its safety and side effects—mainly nervousness, nausea, headaches, and heart palpitations—have scientists concerned.

Since the 1980s, when safe beta-agonists (bronchodilators) became available, the trend has been to use theophylline only after first using the bronchodilators, and then only in resistant cases or to ease nocturnal attacks.

Theophylline can worsen hypertension and may interact with certain drugs such as cimetidine (for heartburn) or erythromycin (for infection). The effective dose of theophylline is very close to the toxic dose. Practitioners at the National Jewish Center, however, state: "Used and monitored properly, under a doctor's care, theophylline remains a safe and useful drug in asthma treatment."

Anticholinergics

Inhaled anticholinergics such as ipratroprium (Atrovent) are the third type of bronchodilator. Atrovent, newly available as an inhalant solution for nebulizers (see p. 129), works by blocking mechanisms that cause muscle contraction, thereby producing relaxation and widening of the airways.

Unlike albuterol, which starts to work in 10–15 minutes, anticholinergics may take 1–3 hours to be effective. Rarely a primary medication, the drug is generally used to prolong the effects of an inhaled beta-agonist or methylxanthine.

Some patients report throat irritation, dry mouth, blurred vision, and difficulty urinating. These side effects suggest that anticholinergics may not be suitable for persons with urinary retention or a tendency to glaucoma.

ANTIHISTAMINES

Although some packages bear the label, "Antihistamines should not be used to treat lower respiratory tract infections, including asthma," current thinking disagrees.

The American Academy of Allergy and Immunology has recommended that the labeling be revised. Antihistamines do relieve symptoms associated with allergic rhinitis, which often leads to asthma. Depending on the dosage, antihistamines can also cause mild bronchodilation, raise the allergen tolerance threshold, and open nasal passages.

With a doctor's approval, allergic asthmatics can tolerate most types of antihistamines used in conjunction with other treatment. Three exceptions are hydroxyzine (Atarax, Vistaril), brompheniramine (Dimetane), and diphenhydramine (Benadryl), which have been reported to cause airway obstruction in a few patients.

For the most part, however, antihistamines as well as specific asthma drugs have taken giant steps in recent years. Try the lowest possible dosage of antihistamines and consider rotating brands to avoid becoming insensitive or overly sensitive. Use them sparingly, cautiously, and wisely.

CHAPTER 14

DON'T YOU BELIEVE IT!

The common denominator in asthma patients is inflamed, hypersensitive airways. Major research is directed at seeking ways to reduce this inflammation, said to be the root of all asthma attacks.

No miracle drug will accomplish this goal, and belief in superstitions, quack remedies, and so-called "natural" cures could keep you from seeking the medical help you may desperately need. That's why it's important to demolish some of the more popular myths about asthma.

MYTH 1:   *Children always outgrow asthma.*

TRUTH: Asthma is the number one cause for hospitalization of children in America. Many seem to outgrow their asthma, but actually, the older they get, the better they learn to prevent and/or control their symptoms. Both children and adults can be asthma-free for years, then get it again.

MYTH 2:   *Asthma isn't as bad as it looks.*

TRUTH: Asthmatics trap 2 liters of air in their chests, the amount of air in a basketball. They can barely breathe. The struggle is frustrating, exhausting, feels terrible, and can be almost as terrifying for onlookers as it is for the patient.

MYTH 3:   *Anyone can use an inhaler. Just put it in your mouth,*
press a button, and breathe in.

TRUTH: Inhalers are the preferred way to take asthma medication. Breathing in delivers the drug directly into the airways,
thus avoiding the systemic side effects of ingesting it. The
method requires use of a metered dose inhaler (MDI) or puffer,
a canister-like gadget with a nozzle at the end. The device looks
simple, but the way to use it has recently changed.

Here's the correct technique:

• Hold inhaler upright, remove cap, and shake.

• Tilt your head slightly back, take a deep breath, exhale.

• Hold the nozzle *one inch* from your open mouth. (Resist the
temptation to close your lips around the mouthpiece. It
causes the medicine to fire directly onto the tongue and
throat, and much less of it reaches the lungs.)

• Press the top to squeeze out a blast of medicine. At the exact
same time, breathe in slowly and deeply through your
mouth.

• Continue breathing in slowly for 3–5 seconds. Avoid quick
gasps.

• Hold your breath 8–10 seconds to let your airways absorb
the medication. Then breathe out slowly.

• Repeat puffs if your doctor has so directed. Wait one minute
between puffs to let the medication penetrate.

• Rinse your mouth with water and spit it out. Don't swallow
the water.

A relatively new device called a spacer or holding chamber
attaches to the canister of the inhaler and holds the medication
until you're ready to inhale it. This allows you to breathe in
more leisurely, helps prevent coughing, and also sifts the medication, trapping the coarser particles and releasing the finer
ones into your lungs. Less of the medicine passes through your

mouth where it could cause *Candida albicans* infection (thrush) or canker sores.

Spacers are available at your pharmacy. Brand names include AeroChamber, Brethancer, and InspirEase.

A recent ban on fluorocarbons, the air-polluting gases used in inhalers, has led to the development of a new type of inhaler. It's an environmentally-friendly breath-activated device that eliminates the need to push down the pump and breathe in at the same moment. One such unit, the Maxair Autohaler, is already on the market.

Some patients, especially children and severe asthmatics, prefer a nebulizer or "breathing machine," which delivers drugs through a face mask. The device pumps compressed air through a solution of liquid medication and produces an extremely fine mist that goes directly to the lungs.

Because nebulizers can deliver a larger dose of medication than inhalers, they tend to cause more side effects.

MYTH 4: *Vitamins and minerals can't help asthma.*

TRUTH: Who knows? Nobel laureate Linus Pauling claimed that vitamin C has a positive effect on allergy-induced asthma, but to date, no scientific evidence bears this out. In reasonable doses, however, vitamin C appears not to be harmful.

The *Journal of the American Dietetic Association* recommends sticking to pills containing simple ascorbic acid. Commercial versions derived from special sources or containing added ingredients claimed to boost the vitamin's absorption only boost the price, not the effectiveness.

Syndicated talk show host Dr. Dean Edell recently reported a study showing that asthma patients who took 100 milligrams of magnesium a day had improved lung function. "But don't run out to the health food store and buy a load of magnesium," he warned. "Get it in a supplement."

MYTH 5: *Asthmatics shouldn't exercise.*

TRUTH: Physical activity is not only possible for asthmatics, it's crucial to good health. In the past, physical exertion was taboo. Asthma patients were told to sit quietly, breathe shallowly, and never strain a muscle.

Today, thanks to new awareness of the mechanics of exercise-related asthma, better drugs, and improved methods of delivering them, exercise is more than encouraged, it's prescribed. At the 1984 Olympics (the last Olympiad for which such figures were kept), 70 athletes had asthma, and 40 of them won medals! The illness has never stopped Jim Ryun or Jackie Joyner-Kersee.

Some of the benefits of exercise are:

- Improved circulation and all the usual advantages of a workout.

- Release of tension.

- Boosted self image.

- Reversal of muscle weakness caused by long-term use of oral steroids.

The keys to a successful program are choosing the right exercises and the best times and places to do them. Heat waves, cold and windy weather, heavily polluted and high pollen days should be avoided.

Low-impact aerobics—walking, jogging, running, biking, working out on machines—are recommended, along with stretching and yoga. Golf and doubles tennis can be beneficial, and hiking and downhill skiing are fine if not too strenuous or done at a high altitude. Wear a face mask to protect your mouth and nose from cold if you ski. Some doctors say swimming is the best exercise of all. If chlorine doesn't bother you, choose heated indoor pools.

Avoid races, tournaments, highly competitive activities, and all contact sports that involve jostling, bumping, pounding, or joint strain. Don't skip warm-ups, and end your exercise gradually.

Check with your doctor before starting any physical routine. Discuss what kind(s) and how much premedication would be right for you. The physician may want you to take an exercise tolerance test in order to evaluate your lung function and capacity. This involves using a stationary bicycle, treadmill, or other machine for about five minutes, or simply running around the office building, then letting the doctor listen to your chest or take a spirometry reading.

Once you begin to exercise, keep your peak flow meter handy so you can monitor your own response. At the first sign of chest tightness or wheezing, stop what you're doing and puff your inhaler. Don't be discouraged by setbacks. Proper exercise can greatly enhance your physical and mental well-being.

MYTH 6:   *Sexual activity should be avoided.*

TRUTH: Many asthmatics fear that the physical exertion of lovemaking will trigger an attack. But good, close, loving sex need not involve acrobatics or be a matter of performance. Sex therapists advise an honest, open relationship with your partner and working together to try different positions that allow easy breathing. Giving up sex can be an added and unnecessary burden.

MYTH 7:   *Breathing exercises are just for children.*

TRUTH: Every asthmatic person can profit from breathing better. When the airways swell and produce excess mucus, less air reaches the lungs and you work harder to breathe.

Most people waste valuable energy by not breathing properly. Never having learned the correct method, they strain chest and neck muscles when they should be using their diaphragm and the muscles between the ribs.

Breathing exercises will help to:

• Increase vital capacity, that is, the amount of air you take in and let out of the lungs.

• Improve gas exchange; oxygen comes in and carbon dioxide goes out.

- Strengthen the correct breathing muscles and increase their effectiveness.
- Train your abdominal muscles to assist your diaphragm in the work of breathing.
- Reduce swelling of the bronchial walls.
- Expel mucus.
- Improve posture.
- Avoid panic and allay fear of suffocation.
- Induce general relaxation and a sense of self-confidence.

For best results, breathing exercises should be done two to four times daily—in the morning before breakfast, during the late afternoon, and/or at night just before going to sleep. Do them at the first hint of a wheeze or a drop in the peak flow meter.

The Asthmatic Children's Foundation in Ossining, New York, suggests several easy exercises. Before starting, remove tight or restrictive clothing and be sure your nasal passages are clear. Then try these:

1. Lie flat with a pillow under your head. Place one hand on your chest (your chest must remain still), the other on your abdomen. Inhale through the nose, feeling your abdomen swell. Pull in your abdomen and exhale through pursed lips, letting out as much air as possible. Repeat 5–10 times.

2. Breathe in normally, then breathe out steadily while blowing through a straw. Place a crumpled paper on a tabletop and see how far you can blow it.

3. Inflate a balloon. Try to get it as large as possible in one breath.

Your doctor or respiratory therapist can personalize the exercises to your specific breathing weaknesses. If you feel tired or dizzy at any time during an exercise, stop immediately and rest.

MYTH 8:   *You can't treat asthma without medication.*

TRUTH: In conjunction with medical care, simple measures can be surprisingly effective. Avoiding allergens is obviously the main goal in allergic asthma, and actions such as keeping pets out of the bedroom or staying indoors during peak pollen hours (usually 5 A.M. to 10 A.M.) can help stave off an attack.

Many doctors recommend the nasal wash—using saline (salt water) irrigation to rinse away mucus and bacteria from the nasal passages. You can buy saline solution at the pharmacy or make it yourself by adding a teaspoon of salt and a pinch of baking soda to a pint of warm water. Pour the solution into the palm of your hand and sniff it up your nose, one nostril at a time. Spit it into the sink, then blow your nose lightly. An eye dropper or an ear syringe can also deliver the saline.

MYTH 9:   *Chicken soup tastes good and feels good but doesn't really do good.*

TRUTH: Hot chicken soup can thin nasal congestion and drain excess mucus, thus helping to clear the airways.

MYTH 10:   *Asthma is caused by stress or emotional problems.*

TRUTH: Make the distinction between cause and trigger. Asthma is a physiological disorder of the airways. It cannot be caused by feelings of guilt, inadequacy, anxiety, or losing a lover. If you have healthy lungs, your response to stress will not be an asthma attack. But an existing lung problem can be aggravated by psychological triggers.

Parents often feel guilty when their children have asthma and tend to blame themselves for a problem they didn't cause. One exception is parents who smoke. Tobacco smoke can be a strong contributing factor in asthma.

MYTH 11:   *Asthma can be very frightening, but never fatal.*

TRUTH: Four thousand Americans die from bronchospasm and asthma-related illnesses every year. However, consistent monitoring with a peak flow meter and learning to recognize the severity of an attack can help prevent fatalities. According to Dr. Tom Plaut, "People don't die because they have asthma. They die because they don't get proper treatment."

MYTH 12: *Foods don't bring on asthma attacks.*

TRUTH: Just as dust, pollens, molds, and pet dander can trigger asthma, so can the foods to which you're allergic. An elimination diet can help pinpoint the offenders, or your doctor can administer a double-blind test in which you swallow capsules of both suspected foods and placebos. The doctor monitors your reaction for several hours with a peak flow meter. Reduced peak flow indicates a possible culprit. Several days of testing may be necessary.

MYTH 13: *Immunotherapy can't help asthma.*

TRUTH: Other than avoidance, immunotherapy in the form of injections is the only nondrug approach to allergic asthma that can lead to long-term relief, possibly even a cure.

Successful treatment with immunotherapy is dependent on knowing exactly what the patient's allergies are. Recent studies with various allergens, especially cat extract, have produced exciting and convincing data that immunotherapy can be very effective.

MYTH 14: *Asthma always leads to emphysema.*

TRUTH: Since asthma symptoms are reversible, they do not necessarily lead to chronic lung disease or even scarred lung tissue.

MYTH 15: *Asthmatics can never lead normal lives.*

TRUTH: This is nonsense. If you are educated and knowledgeable about your illness, if you monitor your peak flow, watch for warning signs and premedicate yourself accordingly, there's no reason you can't enjoy a full, rewarding life.

WARNING: A casual attitude about asthma can be costly to your health. Better to look for triggers, and ways to avoid them, than to rely too heavily on medication.

PART V

MULTIPLE CHEMICAL SENSITIVITY (ENVIRONMENTAL ILLNESS)

In 1985, Janice F., an office assistant to a cardiologist, was working at her desk when a lady patient came in reeking of perfume.

Janice tried to fan the fumes as discreetly as she could, but suddenly she felt herself struggling to breathe. Her heart skipped to 120 beats a minute, twice the normal rate, and her chest felt as if a thick band were constricting it.

Knowing the signs of cardiac arrest, she realized she wasn't having heart problems but rather an asthma attack—serious enough to get herself rushed to the emergency room. There, she was given oxygen and a shot of epinephrine and treated with a nebulizer. After a long night in the hospital, she went home.

Then the problems really started. The moisturizer she had used on her face for years gave her a headache. The detergent she poured into the washing machine launched a sneezing fit. Foods she had eaten all her life with no problem brought on stomach cramps and nausea. Even the ink on her morning newspaper sparked a coughing spree.

That was when Janice realized, to her dismay, that she had become sensitized to everyday chemicals. She had developed multiple chemical sensitivity (MCS)—an illness that the doctor she worked for didn't believe existed.

After experimenting with several allergists and treatments and learning how to keep her environment as "clean" as possible, Janice now has her symptoms somewhat under control. But she had to give up the job she loved, and most likely she won't be able to go back to it.

Janice's case is not untypical. A common scenario is:

1. Patient has a history of allergy, asthma, arthritis, emotional upsets, or other physical or mental conditions that lead to a stressed immune system.

2. Patient has either *chronic low-level chemical exposure*, possibly from office equipment, personal care products, or "sick building" syndrome, or a *one-time high-level exposure*, perhaps from an industrial chemical spill, pesticide spray, new carpeting, or the like.

3. Patient gets asthma or flu-like symptoms and suddenly or gradually begins to react to a wide array of chemical exposures at levels tolerated by most people. Continued low-dose exposure makes symptoms and sensitivity worse.

4. Patient, if lucky, gets an early diagnosis and understands what's happening. Avoidance is the key to recovery.

CHAPTER 15

EPIDEMIC OF THE '90s

Ever since the 1950s when Harvard-trained, board-certified allergist Dr. Theron Randolph first proposed his theory that food allergies could cause a vast range of physical symptoms from bad breath to weight gain, conservative allergists have been challenging his reasoning.

The main contention was use of the word "allergy." The medical establishment had and still has a strict definition: An allergic reaction has to involve the immune system's production of the antibody IgE.

Randolph was unable to provide evidence that the symptoms he saw in special patients were IgE-mediated. When he expanded his theory to include chemical allergies and the whole gamut of emotional ills, he further infuriated conventional allergists. Some doctors tested patients with similar symptoms, found normal levels of IgE, and assumed they were either hysterics or hypochondriacs.

Undeterred, Randolph persisted in his beliefs, claiming that even tiny amounts of chemicals—a whiff of solvent, a pinch of preservative, a dab of petroleum jelly—could provoke a wide range of symptoms. He endorsed the "total load" or allergy threshold concept, likening it to a rain barrel. Everyone has different size barrels, he speculated, filled to various levels. A single drop of water could cause a full barrel to overflow.

As with allergy, an immune system brimming with contaminants from previous chemical exposure would need only a tiny quantity to explode into symptoms. So say the chemically sensitive, who liken themselves to "canaries in the mine shaft." The metaphor dates back to pretechnology days when miners brought live canaries into the caves because the birds were acutely sensitive to dangerous fumes. If a canary became ill or died, the miners knew to avoid the area. MCS patients think they may be human "canaries," warning of a time when much of the civilized world will become chemically ill.

That's only a small part of the controversy sparked by Theron Randolph, a battle that still rages today, as mainstream allergy organizations continue to question the specialty and those who practice it—despite the fact that both sides now agree MCS is not an IgE-mediated allergy. (The mechanism that provokes MCS has yet to be discovered.)

A current position paper from the American Academy of Allergy and Immunology states: "There are no immunologic data to support the dogma of the clinical ecologists. An objective evaluation . . . indicates that it is an unproven and experimental methodology. It is time-consuming and places severe restrictions on the individual's life-style. Individuals being treated in this manner should be fully informed of its experimental nature."

Granted, some practitioners have given clinical ecology a bad name, going to extremes in making wild claims, basing "cures" on severe and unnecessary deprivation, prescribing megadoses of vitamins, recommending quack gadgetry and costly "natural" medication. For this reason, the Society for Clinical Ecology has become the much more respectable-sounding American Academy of Environmental Medicine. (Several organizations with similar names consider MCS a psychiatric illness, so patients should be warned not to seek physician referrals from those societies.)

Also, many medical doctors who used to call themselves clinical ecologists now prefer to be known as environmental specialists, chemical immunologists, environmental allergists, orthomolecular practitioners, and various combinations of those titles.

The point is that MCS does exist. Whether it's an allergy, an "immune system dysregulation" as some advocates claim, a central nervous system disorder, or an altogether different biomedical mechanism not yet understood, the immediate problem is not to define MCS but to try to offer relief to those who suffer it.

TWENTIETH-CENTURY DISEASE

Like the doctors who treat it, MCS has a variety of names: environmental or ecological illness, cerebral allergy, toxic response syndrome, chemical susceptibilities, total allergy syndrome, and more.

Some call it the "twentieth-century disease," attributing the rise of sensitivity to the proliferation of synthetic chemicals after World War II. Other factors are the increase in air and water pollution and the ever-growing number of toxic substances being introduced into our food, clothing, and other products we use daily at home and work.

Many of these products give off gases and particles that have proven toxic in animal and human studies, but few are government- or industry-regulated. We continue using them because they're there—and because most people get away with minor or no symptoms. Others aren't so lucky. They become ill from eating, touching, inhaling, or absorbing small amounts of widely used "safe" chemicals. Reactions can be immediate or delayed and range from mild irritation to major disability.

These symptoms perplex many doctors, especially psychiatrists, some of whom have become serious obstacles to research and action. The majority, untrained to recognize MCS, tend to brand this illness as paranoia, panic disorder, or hysteria.

Because of the stigmatization and financial difficulties associated with such debilitating symptoms, many MCS patients do suffer depression and emotional problems, but to conclude that MCS is psychogenic (mental in origin) would be unscientific and irresponsible.

Not to be underestimated are the public relations and legal battles waged by health insurance companies and other vested forces who don't want to have to accept liability and pay disability benefits, industrial giants unwilling to take on the burden of workers' complaints or the cost of changing technology, and the staggering number of manufacturers who produce low-level chemical products.

As evidence and case histories accumulate, however, the diagnosis of MCS appears to be heading toward wider acceptance. Even the federal government is showing some interest—with good reason.

GULF WAR SYNDROME

An estimated 30,000 to 50,000 (out of 570,000) Desert Storm veterans, heroes of America's most recent war, have come home to experience a distressing array of ailments with no apparent cause.

Environmental illness experts who have studied the situation believe the symptoms point directly to a diagnosis of MCS. They cite the situation overseas: Military personnel were given numerous inoculations to protect against biological and chemical warfare agents. Their uniforms were impregnated with insecticide, and they were in constant proximity to pesticides (including DDT), fumes from tank exhaust, burning oil wells, garbage heaps, and production plants, as well as severe industrial pollution from neighboring cities. Add to this the intense stress of war and an epidemic of bites from parasite-infected sand flies, and you have the kind of triggers many MCS patients believe set off their own symptoms.

Clearly, these Gulf War veterans were exposed to extremely high levels of chemicals for which they're now paying a huge price. To worsen matters, well-intentioned doctors, not knowing what else to do, have overdosed the returned vets with pain-killers, antidepressants, and antibiotics.

"Three characteristics of this illness point directly and un-questionably to MCS," states Major Richard Haines, a Vietnam vet who was not in the Persian Gulf himself, but saw so many men in his battalion return sick, he began his own investigation.

"One is the delayed symptomatology. With chemicals, organ damage usually doesn't show up till six to twelve months later in the form of liver dysfunction, immune system depression, thyroid and other problems. Two is the fact it's a multisystem disorder, and three is the widespread allergic sensitivity to foods and traditional allergens."

On his own time, with his own money, Haines formed an enormous data base of facts and addresses from mailed-in ques-tionnaires. What he learned was this:

- Twenty-seven out of 28 Gulf vets tested showed a sensitivity to low levels of everyday chemicals.

- The average sick vet has 20–30 symptoms that make it diffi-cult or impossible for him or her to work.

- The most common complaints are headaches, sore joints, fa-tigue, disturbed vision, memory and concentration loss, stomach upset, fungus infections (*Candida*, especially in the mouth), and a white, scaly foot rash.

- Those who showed no improvement either smoke or work in a contaminated environment. That includes foundries, plating plants, most factories, and situations that involve plastics or man-made synthetics.

"The real nightmare," Haines continues, "are the Gulf War babies. They're having allergies and reacting negatively to baby formula, food, and medication. We're also seeing a lot of defor-mities and immune depression. The situation is far worse than anyone knows."

MCS appears to afflict mainly well-educated middle-aged white females, but along with the babies, males of all ages, races, and backgrounds have also become victims.

Despite the medical community's divisiveness over the issue, press attention and public indignation have motivated some government action. At present, four federal agencies—the Social Security Administration, the U.S. Department of Housing and Urban Development (HUD), the U.S. Department of Education, and the Civil Rights Division of the U.S. Department of Justice—have officially recognized chemical sensitivity as a disability. Much more government recognition, however, is needed.

According to Earon Davis, J.D., M.P.H., legal adviser to the National Center for Environmental Health Strategies (NCEHS), "It is easier for those who may be morally and/or financially responsible for these disabling illnesses to deny that chemical sensitivity is a proven illness. In this way, they can imply that the problem is psychosomatic . . . to escape the consequences of their poor judgment."

Adds Mary Lamielle, president of NCEHS: "Our war heroes deserve dignity, compassion and open minds. The burden of proof must not be borne by these disabled veterans."

People who want information or think they may be a victim of Gulf War syndrome may call Richard Haines' Desert Storm Vets 24-hour hotline at 812-948-9366, or the Desert Storm Veterans Coalition at 800-307-1330.

CHAPTER 16

ARE YOU A CANDIDATE?

Several years ago, I sat in the office of the late Dr. Phyllis Saifer, a brilliant allergist who suffered from MCS and did much to foster understanding of the illness. I watched as her technician gave a double-blind provocation test to a young woman. The first four times drops were squirted under the woman's tongue, she showed no reaction, sitting quietly and calmly. The fifth time, she began to shift in her chair, obviously distressed. She blew her nose, rubbed her eyes, and began to weep.

I later learned the first four doses were placebos; the fifth was a chemical. Nothing was staged for my benefit. I just happened to be present, being skin-tested for conventional allergies. But what I saw made me a believer. I remain convinced that chemicals can trigger depression and emotional reactions as well as an almost unlimited range of physical symptoms.

MCS is, in fact, a multiple organ system disorder that affects many different organs in various parts of the body. One can sympathize with a doctor presented with such a bewildering array of symptoms. Is rapid heartbeat a cardiac problem or a reaction to cigar smoke? Is a headache signaling a brain tumor or a food allergy? Are the two complaints related?

Because MCS is a new disease and still widely misunderstood, few diagnostic tests are as reliable as self-observation. If you think you may be chemically sensitive, ask yourself these questions:

1. Do gas stations make you feel queasy or strange?

2. Does perfume give you any unpleasant feelings?

3. Have you ever been to a park or open field and suffered headaches or other symptoms, then later learned the area had recently been sprayed?

4. Have you ever felt faint or dizzy in a beauty or hair salon?

5. Do you react to a bathroom that smells of disinfectant?

6. Have you ever walked into a pharmacy or department store, felt confused, and wondered why you were there?

7. Do specific foods make you feel ill?

8. Does the exhaust of cars or buses bother you?

9. Have you ever felt "spacy" in an airplane, an office, or an energy-tight building?

10. Does the smell of certain products make you nauseated?

If you answered yes to one or more questions, you may be slightly chemically sensitive and in danger of "overflowing the barrel." Seemingly minor symptoms can be valuable warning signs. Start immediately to cut down your exposure to chemicals (see Chapter 17), and don't become a candidate for MCS.

WHO'S AT RISK

A number of researchers have sought to determine which groups of people are most vulnerable to MCS. The only common denominator they found was chemical exposure, either a one-time major blast or a chronic low-level infusion. Socioeconomic, racial, and cultural backgrounds matter little except that the wealthy have more options for avoidance.

Those at high risk include:

- People who work in energy-sealed buildings and breathe fumes from construction materials, office equipment, and disinfectants, along with tobacco smoke and other inhalants.

- People who live in energy-tight homes and breathe fumes from carpets, consumer products, pesticides, and household cleaners as well as airborne allergens.

- Factory workers who handle industrial chemicals, especially in plants that process wood, metal, plastics, paints, and textiles.

- Agricultural workers in constant contact with pesticides, fungicides, and fertilizer full of bacteria and allergens.

- People who live in high-pollution areas.

- People in specific occupations such as dry cleaning, hairdressing and makeup, pest control, printing, photocopying, aerospace, and computers.

- The unborn children of these people.

Other contributing factors are youth, old age, chronic illness, malnutrition, poverty, a history of allergy, and a stressful, high-risk occupation.

DIAGNOSIS

A diagnosis of MCS is generally made (1) on the basis of the patient's history and (2) after a doctor has excluded all other possible diagnoses. The combination of these two factors may lead the doctor to order testing.

Gunnar Heuser, M.D., a Los Angeles immunologist and toxicologist, uses a SPECT (single photon emission computed tomography) scan to monitor MCS patients while he challenges them with a low dose of a chemical such as chlorine. The sophisticated test uses radioactive gas to create a color image showing the flow of blood that supplies the brain with oxygen. In most chemically injured patients, there's a definite decrease in blood flow to the brain, corresponding with their complaints of confusion, memory loss, headaches, fatigue, and poor concentration.

Other tests favored by environmental specialists are provocative-neutralization (P-N) and serial titration.

P-N can be sublingual, intradermal, or (less commonly) inhaled or swallowed. The technique is used to provoke symptoms by controlled exposure to the suspected substance for diagnostic purposes (provocation) and then to relieve symptoms (neutralization).

Here's how P-N works: The technician delivers a diluted extract of substance X, the test substance, under the tongue or skin. If symptoms develop, the assumption is that substance X caused the reaction. That's the provocation dose. Decreasing doses are then administered until symptoms disappear. That's the neutralization dose. The patient takes home a small bottle of the neutralizing dose to use sublingually when reactions occur.

Over a period of time, probably one or two years, frequency of use can be reduced as symptoms lessen. Some patients remain symptom-free on a maintenance regime of one or two doses a week. Others heal sufficiently to stop taking the extracts entirely.

Why or how P-N works no one seems to know. Circumstantial evidence indicates that it does work in many cases, but in a recent University of California study, saltwater injections relieved symptoms as effectively as the neutralizing dose.

Somewhat less controversial is serial titration, generally an intradermal test using progressively weaker or stronger dilutions of substance X to determine the "end point"—the weakest dilution that produces a reaction. This supplies diagnostic information and the starting dosage for immunotherapy injections or sublingual drop treatment.

The lack of reliable diagnostic tests may be one reason MCS has not been better accepted by mainstream medicine. Nevertheless, there are other routes to diagnosis.

SYMPTOMS

People like to say it's easier to list the symptoms that are not associated with MCS than to list the ones that are. Certain body disruptions, however, seem to appear more frequently than others. These are characteristic of MCS:

EYES

Bags, dark circles under eyes
Double, blurred, or distorted vision
Drooping or red eyelids
Inability to tolerate fluorescent light
Inflammation
Itching, watering, or burning
Swelling around eyes

EARS

Dizziness, imbalance
Itching, aching, feeling of fullness
Loss of hearing
Ringing, popping
Sensitivity to noise
Throbbing

NOSE

Bleeding
Frequent colds, flu-like syndrome
Increased sense of smell
Itching, sneezing
Loss of sense of smell
Postnasal drip
Watery discharge and congestion

MOUTH

Burning tongue
Canker sores

Dryness

Metallic taste

THROAT

Cough

Itchy palate

Soreness, dryness, hoarseness

LUNGS

Asthma

Difficult breathing ("air hunger")

Rapid breathing

Wheezing

CARDIOVASCULAR

Chest pains, tightening

Flushing, chills

Rapid, pounding, or irregular heartbeat

Redness or blueness of hands and feet

CENTRAL NERVOUS SYSTEM

Anxiety, irritability

Aphasia (inability to speak or comprehend language)

"Brain fatigue" or weary brain

Chronic fatigue

Confusion or disorientation

Depression

Fainting

Headache, migraine

Hyperactivity, overstimulation

Impaired motor control

Mood swings

Poor concentration

Seizures

Short-term memory loss

Sleep disturbances

Spacy, floating feeling

(Extreme reactions can cause delusions, hallucinations, amnesia, psychosis)

GASTROINTESTINAL

Alcohol intolerance

Bloating

Burning

Constipation

Cramps

Diarrhea

Excessive thirst

Food intolerances; indigestion, heartburn

Gastroenteritis (inflammation of stomach and intestine)

Nausea, vomiting

Upset stomach

GENITOURINARY

Abnormal or irregular menstrual periods

Blood in urine

Frequent or painful urination

Impotence

Itching or burning rectum

Vaginal itching or discharge

MUSCULOSKELETAL

Backaches

Joint and muscle pains

Lack of coordination

Muscle spasms

Muscle weakness

"Restless legs"

Swollen limbs

SKIN
_____

Acne
Flushing, burning, tingling
Hives, blisters, rashes
Itching
Sensitive skin
Sweating at back of neck
_____

If you've been bothered by any or many of the preceding ailments, you don't necessarily have MCS. But your symptoms may be MCS-related if:

- Your doctor(s) can find no other reason for them after thorough examination and testing.

- You have a history of allergy, asthma, arthritis, or auto-immune disease.

- They change. One day you have sore joints, the next day a headache.

- They come and go intermittently.

- They get worse with physical activity or exercise.

- They seem to be greater on one side of the body.

- They heal rapidly or not at all.

- Minor stresses trigger major aches.

- You can't tolerate most medication.

- You gain or lose weight without trying.

- You feel helpless, frustrated, angry, and depressed.

Now that you've gathered a collection of data about yourself, write down all related observations: where and when you get symptoms, products you suspect, where you feel the best or worst, and so on. Take them to a reputable doctor who specializes in environmental illness. Even though MCS is not, by strict definition, an allergy, it behaves like one in many ways, and the environmental specialists who treat it are usually allergists.

HOW TO FIND A SPECIALIST

Connecting with the right doctor is not as difficult as it sounds. Susan Springer, former president of the Environmental Health Network (EHN), suggests you first write to the American Academy of Environmental Medicine in Denver (see Appendix B).

"They'll send a referral list of doctors in your area who are sensitive to MCS," she says. "It's also a good idea to contact the major national organizations: The Chemical Injury Information Network, the Human Ecology Action League, the National Center for Environmental Health Strategies, and the EHN [see Appendix B]. They all have newsletters that are pretty interactive. People write in about their experiences with doctors and treatments.

"You might want to join a support group or get peer counseling," she adds. "Quite a few doctors have made tapes you can buy or listen to. Many people log onto computer networks through disability and chronic illness conferences. The best way to find a doctor is to get names and input from as many people as possible." (See Chapter 4.)

Joining a national organization such as the EHN is wise advice. You not only feel less alone with your problem, you're exposed to experts in the field, and you'll have access to information about the latest medical, political, legal, and financial ramifications of MCS.

CHAPTER 17

WAKE UP AND SMELL THE CHEMICALS

With your new knowledge and awareness, the world around you will begin to look quite different—even your own home. Familiar products such as perfume and after-shave may suddenly loom threatening and, depending on your degree of sensitivity, should probably be replaced, especially if you develop respiratory problems or asthma.

Unless you're seriously ill, however, don't go to extremes. Ignore fanatics who insist your only hope for survival is to pack up and move to the mountains. Instead, focus your efforts on cleaning up the environment where you spend two-thirds of your time. Start with making your bedroom an oasis. Remove suspected agents one or two at a time and check results.

Here are some general guidelines for the home:

- Don't smoke in your home and don't allow anyone else to do so.

- As gradually as you like, replace toxic products with non-toxic or substitute products (see next section). The first items to consider should be:

  - Aerosol sprays
  - Air fresheners/deodorizers
  - Chlorinated water

- Dry-cleaned clothes and draperies
- Felt-tip pens
- Furniture and floor polish
- Gas stoves and appliances
- Glues, adhesives
- Household cleaners, bleaches, detergents, and disinfectants
- Kerosene heaters
- Mothballs
- Nail polish and remover
- Newsprint with fresh ink
- Paint supplies and varnish
- Pesticides and fungicides
- Pliable plastics such as mattress covers, shower curtains, tablecloths, and food wrap (hard plastics, such as telephones, emit fewer fumes)
- Rubbing alcohol
- Scented products such as soaps, shampoos, cosmetics, and deodorants
- Stain removers and stain-proofers
- Synthetic fabrics and permanent-press clothing

- Take all your old or unused chemical products, including paints and cleaning supplies, to a hazardous waste disposal center.
- Don't buy any products with such strongly worded warnings as "poisonous," "toxic," "dangerous when inhaled," or "use in a well-ventilated area."
- Check labels! Many products contain VOCs—volatile organic compounds—meaning that they mix with the air you breathe and can emit potentially harmful gases. But don't count on labels to tell everything. Nothing in your bedroom warns that your new set of cabinets may be releasing low levels of formaldehyde fumes.

- *Consumer Reports* lists six solvents to "be used with great caution." Better still, avoid them if you can:
  - *Methylene chloride*—found in degreasers, waxes, paint products, pesticides, lubricants.
  - *Toluene*—found in gasoline, some glues, paint products, nail polishes.
  - *1,1,1 Trichloroethane*—found in drain cleaners, spot removers, shoe polish, insecticides, printing inks, degreasers.
  - *Glycol ethers*—found in antifreeze, some paints, adhesives, sealants.
  - *N-Hexane*—found in glues, paints, varnishes, printing inks.
  - *Petroleum distillates* (including benzene)—found in a wide array of products: pesticides, paints, furniture polish, adhesives, spot removers, caulking compounds, detergents.

  Temporary exposure to VOCs can cause drowsiness, dizziness, headache, breathing difficulty, and eye irritation. Long-term exposure can affect the nervous, respiratory, and reproductive systems, liver, heart, and kidneys. Cancer and birth defects have also been reported.

- If you must use a solvent for any reason, take precautions. Don't use more than one at a time, and don't drink alcoholic beverages that day because they can increase the toxic effects. Ask your doctor about interactions with medication. Wear a respirator (a nose mask sold in paint shops and safety equipment supply stores), gloves, and goggles, and try to work standing up. Chemical fumes tend to sink.

- Open windows as much as possible and install exhaust fans to increase ventilation. Keep windows closed if you live in a high-pollution area or on a heavily traveled street full of car exhaust fumes. Consider adding a high-quality air filter (see Chapter 8).

- Don't use unvented gas, oil, or wood heaters, and don't idle your motor when the car is in the garage. Carbon monoxide can cause nausea, dizziness, and disorientation.

- Test your home for radon, a colorless, odorless radioactive gas that may, with prolonged exposure to high levels, increase the risk of lung cancer. Call the EPA Radon Hotline, 800-SOS-RADON, for an information kit.

SAFE SUBSTITUTES

Americans have become obsessed with smelling good. No mannerly person would dare to perspire noticeably at a party or exhale garlic fumes at the office. Madison Avenue spends billions programming us to buy sweet-scented preparations to mask body odors when we'd be far healthier smelling like ourselves.

Similarly, our homes are expected to be almost as sterile as our bodies. We dump blue liquids into our toilets, bleach our clothes, spray pine-scented chemicals into the air, and spritz our garbage cans with lemon mist. To what end? The air we take into our lungs becomes further contaminated.

Six nontoxic household products, used correctly, can replace almost all commercial cleaners and deodorizers. One or more are probably already in your kitchen. You'll find them less costly, easier to apply, and far gentler on your hands, your body, and the atmosphere. They are:

Baking Soda

Sodium bicarbonate cleans, removes spots, softens water, deodorizes, and can be used dry as an underarm deodorant. May be sprinkled on rugs before vacuuming.

Borax

Sodium borate acts as a general disinfectant, whitens and brightens laundry, cleans bathrooms and garbage cans, freshens carpets, and can replace scouring cleanser. Call the Dial Consumer Information Center (the Dial Corp. makes Borax) at 800-457-8739 for a list of tested and recommended uses. Caution: Keep away from children.

Soap

Pure fragrance-free soap is not made with petroleum derivatives and is biodegradable (capable of decomposing).

Washing Soda

Hydrated (combined with water) sodium carbonate cuts grease, removes stains, disinfects, and softens water. Most supermarkets carry sal soda, as it's also called, in the laundry section. Be sure it's not scented.

White Vinegar

A versatile disinfectant. Dilute with equal parts water to clean tile and formica and to remove spots, molds, mineral deposits, and crayon marks. Combine with salt to clean copper and brass.

Lemon Juice

Use as vinegar when a fresh scent is desired. Also cleans copper and brass.

The six agents listed above should meet all your housecleaning needs. Now try a few "recipes":

AIR FRESHENER. Set out a bottle of vanilla extract, boil cloves or cinnamon in water, or drop a half lemon into your garbage disposal unit. Open containers of baking soda or white vinegar will absorb odors.

DEER, RABBIT, GOPHER REPELLENT. Human hair (get clippings from a barber or beauty shop) in a mesh bag will repel most garden invaders. Sprinkle red pepper or talcum powder at the base of plants to keep rabbits away.

DISINFECTANT. Mix ½ cup borax with a gallon of hot water. A California hospital tested this mix and found it met all germicide requirements.

DRAIN CLEANER. Pour ½ cup baking soda into the drain, add a cup of water and a cup of white vinegar. Wait about 10 minutes while it foams, then flush with plenty of hot water.

FLEA REPELLENT FOR PETS. Add 1 teaspoon vinegar to a quart of water and pour on pet. Keep fur brushed and clean.

FURNITURE POLISH. Apply lemon or olive oil. Sprinkle a little cornstarch and rub to a shine.

GLASS CLEANER. Mix ½ cup white vinegar with 2 cups warm water. Use week-old newspapers to polish.

INSECTICIDE. Add 2–3 drops of dishwashing liquid to a quart of water and spray plants with mixture once a month.

INSECT REPELLENT. Rub vanilla extract on your skin. Or crush bay leaves in your fingers, then rub fingers over your skin. (Good for mosquitoes, gnats, flies.)

LAUNDRY CLEANER. Grate pure bar soap, add water, liquefy in blender. For heavy stains, add borax and washing soda to washing machine.

MOTH REPELLENT. NEVER use mothballs. Seal clothes in zipper bags. Or mix 2 parts mint, 1 part thyme, and 1 part cloves and hang in a cheesecloth bag in your closet.

OVEN CLEANER. Use aluminum foil to catch juices. Pour salt on soiled area before oven cools, then clean with baking soda and water.

PESTICIDE. Keep area spotlessly clean, especially hard-to-reach places. Try natural pest control. Repel ants by sealing points of entry with toothpaste, caulk, or tape. Drive them from the kitchen by sprinkling borax, chili pepper, cinnamon, cloves, or baking soda on shelves and counters and into crevices. Repeat often.

Keep ants from pet food by putting the dog or cat bowl in another shallow bowl with an inch or so of water around it.

To trap roaches, put a small chunk of banana and some bacon grease into a 4-inch-high glass jar. Spread a 1-inch layer of Vaseline around the jar ½ inch from the top. To repel roaches, use bay leaves or cucumber rinds.

Repair all kitchen leaks and cracks, and don't leave any food sitting out or bits of food on unwashed dishes. Cover the soil around the house with diatomaceous earth, a light-colored porous rock sold in garden supply stores. For further information, call the National Pesticide Telecommunications Network sponsored by the EPA: 800-858-PEST.

SILVER CLEANER. Rub silver gently with toothpaste on a wet cloth or a mixture of baking soda and water. Use olive oil to clean pewter.

SPOT REMOVER. Use club soda or a mix of half white vinegar, half water.

FORMALDEHYDE

So much has been written about formaldehyde and its potential to cause neurological damage and cancer, it warrants a section of its own. Formaldehyde is a colorless, strong-smelling (in large concentrations) gas that affects people differently.

Some react to it as an irritant, experiencing burning sensations in the eyes, nose, and throat. Others develop allergic skin reactions through physical contact with such products as durable-press clothing, or they wheeze and become asthmatic after inhaling fumes. Most people, however, don't react at all to common low-level exposures.

Whether the level in your home is high or low depends mainly on what's releasing the gas, the amount of ventilation, the temperature, and humidity. Higher temperatures and humidity increase emissions, and new products outgas (release gas) more frequently than older ones.

Major sources of formaldehyde in the home are:

1. Burning materials such as wood, kerosene, cigarettes, and natural gas.

2. Carpets. They trap formaldehyde emitted from other sources and release it when temperature and humidity rise.

3. Cosmetics, paints, glues, coated paper products.

4. Permanent-press fabrics and draperies and other synthetic textiles.

5. Pressed wood products such as particleboard (sheet material made of wood fragments bonded with resin), plywood, and medium-density fiberboard, which are used to make shelves, kitchen cabinets, and furniture.

6. Urea-formaldehyde foam insulation (UFFI). In the save-energy frenzy of the 1970s, many homes installed UFFI and many occupants became ill. The foam outgases heavily when new, but the effect diminishes after about five years.

Some ways to reduce formaldehyde exposure are by washing permanent-press fabrics before wearing them, using air conditioning to keep the temperature cool and to lower humidity, using a dehumidifier in wet climates, removing or replacing known sources, and letting large amounts of fresh air into the home or office.

For further information, call the EPA Toxic Substance Control Act assistance line: 202-554-1404.

COSMETICS AND BEAUTY PRODUCTS

The FDA does not pass approval on cosmetics, but does require a listing of ingredients. The burden then falls on you to read the labels and look for possible allergens and irritants. Any cosmetic that has a warning label should be discarded.

Here are some ingredients to look for. Use them minimally or avoid:

Acetone

Found in nail polish remover. Can cause nail-splitting and skin rashes. Inhalation may irritate lungs.

Benzalkonium Chloride (BAK)

Found in after-shave products, hair tonics, eye lotions. Can cause allergic conjunctivitis.

Bithionol

Found in cold creams, moisturizers, hair preparations, after-shave lotions, and medicated cosmetics. Causes photosensitivity (sensitivity to light) and skin rashes.

Blue Dye No. 1

Found in after-shave lotions, toothpastes, blushes, purple lipsticks. Suspected carcinogen.

Butylated Hydroxytoluene (BHT)

Found in baby oils, soaps, eyeliner pencils. Corrosive to skin, can cause allergy.

Coal Tar

Found in cosmetic dyes. Potent allergen, causes cancer in animals.

Dimethyl Sulfate

Found in dyes and perfumes. Vapors hurt the eyes. Sufficient skin absorption can cause serious poisoning.

Formaldehyde

Found in deodorants, toothpaste, mouthwashes, shampoos, hair-setting lotions, nail polish, perfumes, bath tissues. May cause peeling nails, skin rashes, eye and respiratory tract irritation. A frequent sensitizer.

Green Dye No. 6

Found in pine shampoos, mint toothpastes. Possible carcinogen.

Iron Oxides

Found in eye makeup, lipsticks, rouge. Suspected carcinogen.

Lead Acetate

Found in hair dyes, face creams. A proven carcinogen; may cause lead buildup.

Perfume

A frequent allergen, found in every type of cosmetic. Can cause headaches, dizziness, skin rashes, coughing, and vomiting.

Phenylenediamine

Found in hair dyes. May produce eczema, bronchial asthma, gastritis, skin rash.

Polyvinylpyrrolidone (PVP)

Found in eyeliners, hair sprays, hair-setting gels, rouge. May cause lung damage.

Toluene

Found in nail polish. Can cause liver damage, irritation to skin and respiratory tract.

Triethanolomine (TEA)

Found in moisturizing creams, suntan lotions, hair gels. Toxic effect on animals.

The main problem with cosmetics is that if a product seems to work, people tend to stick to it, use it daily or several times a day, and become dependent on it. Overuse, as with almost any substance, can lead to developing a sensitivity.

You can avoid the problem by rotating your usual cosmetics with safe alternatives. Try these suggestions:

AFTER-SHAVE. Use rubbing alcohol, diluted lemon juice, or diluted mint flavoring.

BATH POWDER. Try cornstarch, if you're not allergic to corn.

DEODORANT. Use baking soda or vinegar. (The smell disappears as it dries.)

EYELINER. Try charcoal from a wood fire on a Q-tip. Avoid ashes and keep eye closed as you apply it.

EYE DROPS. Place cucumber slices or wet tea bags on closed eyes and leave in place for at least five minutes.

HAIR CONDITIONER. Beat an egg, apply to wet, washed hair, rinse thoroughly.

MOISTURIZER. Try canola, olive, or any light cooking oil.

MOUTHWASH. Try cooled mint tea or ½ teaspoon baking soda in a cup of water.

SHAVING CREAM. Soak skin with hot wash cloth, leave cloth in place while skin softens. Use electric razor.

TOOTHPASTE. Use baking soda or an electric toothbrush with water. (It's the brushing that loosens food debris, not the toothpaste.)

AT THE OFFICE

You have a right to breathe clean air where you work, even though your co-workers may get irritated at having to walk a few more steps to the copy machine, being asked not to wear cologne, or having to leave the building to smoke.

The same principles apply to the office as to the home, but

controlling a work situation isn't always possible. Emissions from supplies and equipment can be significant, leading to such complications as "laser printer rhinitis," hoarseness from carbonless paper, and asthma and breathing difficulties from ozone released by copiers.

The good news is that major companies are aware of the problem, and most are seeking to remedy it. Microsoft's Windows, for example, makes it possible to place a computer in a vented glass case and enter data with a pointing device such as a mouse. This allows physical distance from the machine and its vapors.

Even better news is that "healthy building" is becoming almost as familiar a term as "sick building." In San Francisco, for example, national attention has focused on the new Main Library structure due for completion in 1996.

Working with an air-quality consultant, architects are placing photocopiers in separate uncarpeted rooms with their own exhaust system, so that chemical fumes will not enter the rest of the building. No particleboard will be used, special low-emission carpets have been developed, and engineers have made certain that large quantities of outside air will flow through the halls. Doors will open onto terraces, and staff lounge windows will be operable.

Enthusiasts hope San Francisco's Main Library will inspire similar buildings across the nation.

Mary Lamielle, dynamic president of the National Center for Environmental Health Strategies, suggests that every chemically sensitive person should be entitled to:

- An office with a window that opens and adequate ventilation.

- An environment free of tobacco smoke, pesticides, air fresheners, disinfectants, fragrance-laden cleaning products, and exhaust fumes from the parking garage.

- Furnishings and supplies that are the least toxic or allergenic.

- Prenotification of painting, remodeling, or pesticide application, with provisions for alternate work arrangements.
- Education of co-workers about MCS to avert stigma, harassment, and discrimination.
- Options to work at peak ventilation periods.
- When feasible, the option to work at home.

Remember that your employer is required by law to ensure that you have safe working conditions, adequate training, and whatever protective gear you may need.

Become familiar with your workplace rights. You may be entitled to "reasonable accommodation" under the Americans with Disabilities Act (ADA). Check your state labor or industrial relations department for access to OSHA and NIOSH (National Institute for Occupational Safety and Health). They may have vital information about your specific workplace problems.

TRAVEL TIPS

Traveling can be hazardous to your health if you're chemically sensitive. Enclosed quarters on buses, trains, planes, and ship cabins leave you little escape from cosmetic, clothing, and grooming scents of fellow passengers. Windows of buses and trains let in potent diesel fumes, and airplanes often reek of pesticides, but the open deck of an ocean liner offers some of the cleanest air to be found.

If you prefer driving, choose a broken-in older car whose "new" smell has long evaporated. A small, lightweight auto uses less gas, and its front seat should be sufficiently distant from exhaust fumes. Look for uncrowded highways and mountain and coast routes. Stay far from freeways, industrial centers, and newly sprayed farmlands.

Try to settle into a country inn or a large, older hotel rather than a new, modern one. Bring your own shampoo and baking soda or Bon Ami cleanser for the bathroom. (Special products for allergic/sensitive travelers are available from many companies listed in Appendix D.)

Be sure to ask about an EverGreen room. Hotels and motels in 13 states—Alabama, Arizona, Arkansas, California, Florida, Georgia, Kentucky, Louisiana, Mississippi, North Carolina, South Carolina, Tennessee, and Texas—now have set aside rooms that feature smoke-free, odor-free, allergen-free air and a filtered drinking water system. Call EverGreen Room Properties for more details: 800-929-2626, weekdays, 9 A.M. to 5 P.M. EST.

When booking a room, don't be afraid to phone ahead and ask the housekeeper:

1. Has the hotel recently been sprayed with pesticides, painted, or remodeled? (If yes, stay elsewhere.)

2. Do you have a room with a window that opens and/or a balcony? (Make sure it's away from the chlorinated swimming pool.)

3. Do you have a room on the top floor? (The higher you go, the cleaner the air.)

4. Is it possible to get a room that has not been newly cleaned with disinfectant or strong-smelling cleanser?

5. Could you remove all soaps, shampoos, air fresheners, and similar products and open the window (away from the swimming pool) several hours before I arrive?

With luck and careful planning, the majority of your symptoms may vanish in a vacation hideaway, and shed some light on the culprits you left behind.

CHAPTER 18

GETTING WELL

If you're lucky enough to find the right doctor and have your illness properly diagnosed, you may be offered several options for treatment (in addition to avoidance.)

One is to start a doctor-approved multivitamin and mineral regimen to boost energy. Pills without additives or fillers are available in most health food stores. B-vitamins, especially, should be free of yeast, soy, and dairy products.

Another option is to make the necessary dietary changes if you haven't already done so (see Chapters 10 and 11). Chemically sensitive persons tend to be allergic to a wide variety of foods.

Depending on your degree of chemical sensitivity, you may want to add several test substances to the basic food elimination diet. Try challenging yourself by eliminating and later reintroducing the following:

• Tap water in a glass container. Drinking water tends to be heavily treated with chemicals.

• Distilled water in a plastic container. If you get symptoms, consider the plastic.

• Food (to which you're not allergic) that comes wrapped in plastic.

• Any vegetable to which you're not allergic, in these forms: fresh organic, fresh nonorganic, canned, and frozen.

While not terribly accurate, these additions to the basic food elimination diet may give you some idea of the degree of your chemical sensitivity. If pesticide-free peas trouble you less than supermarket peas, buy organic. If foods or drinks exposed to plastic wrap seem to make you feel worse, try eliminating anything plastic-wrapped for three weeks, then challenge yourself again.

Do the same for foods in cans. You may be responding to the phenol lining of cans. In all cases, be sure you're reacting to the container and not the contents.

At the same time, follow these general diet rules:

1. *Stick to low-fat foods.* Skim milk has as many nutrients as homogenized. Choose lean cuts of meat and trim all fat, because that's where pesticides accumulate. Remove skin from poultry. Bake, broil, or stew fish, meats, and poultry instead of frying them.

1. *Cook stews and soups a day in advance,* refrigerate, and skim off fat.

2. *Limit sodium* by using fresh herbs, olive oil, and lemon juice to replace high-salt seasonings such as soy sauce, catsup, and prepared salad dressings.

3. *Choose brown rice and whole-grains* instead of white rice and "enriched" white bread.

4. *Eat fresh fruits and vegetables.* Natural flavors of vegetables steamed in the microwave can be delicious if you train your palate to appreciate them. Try asparagus, summer squash, broccoli.

Procter & Gamble is currently promoting Fit Produce Rinse, a cleanser claimed to remove 70 percent of surface wax, dirt, and chemicals from fresh produce. Other alternatives are to carefully wash produce yourself, peel or discard the outsides, buy organic foods grown without pesticides, or choose roots—carrots, potatoes, beets, onions, and the like—which have not been overly sprayed. You might even enjoying growing your own produce.

5. *Read labels!* Some are irrelevant. One package of frozen broccoli, for instance, boasts, "No added salt, sugar, or cholesterol. No preservatives." Big deal. Other labels can be blatantly deceptive. Products claiming "No artificial preservatives" are often full of *real* preservatives.

6. *Rotate the foods you eat.* The more varied your diet, the less your chances of reacting.

LIFESTYLES

Adjustments in living habits are as vital as dietary changes. If the previously suggested avoidance measures aren't enough to decrease your total load of toxins, you may want to consider a detox clinic.

Programs for MCS patients can include sweating out chemicals through saunas, exercises, and chelation therapy, a controversial technique for extracting heavy metals from the body. Massage, immunotherapy, psychological and nutritional counseling may also be offered.

A word of warning: Quackery and fake "cures" abound for this illness. MCS patients are often misunderstood, depressed, and desperate—ideal marks for unscrupulous hustlers. Do not sign up for any treatment or enter any detox program without first checking its medical staff, equipment, costs, and reputation. Try to question former patients. That advice cannot be too strongly emphasized.

Check also for insurance reimbursement. Some programs are approved for persons chemically injured on the job—for example, firemen, pest exterminators, pesticide sprayers, even blue- and white-collar workers who have had toxic exposure.

Perhaps the best known reputable clinic is Dr. William Rea's Environmental Health Center, a medical facility in Dallas, Texas, with a staff of 60. Founded in 1974, the clinic claims to provide an "environmentally safe" setting designed to exclude "all the obvious sources of offending substances." Furniture is made of natural materials, walls are porcelain steel (steel that has been fired with a vitreous coating), floors are tile, and the water and ventilation systems are carefully filtered.

Services include a complete medical exam, blood and skin tests, nutritional counseling, cardiovascular fitness testing, psychological counseling, biofeedback and stress management, a detoxification program, and immunotherapy.

Patients pay $4,500 a month plus $40 a night for nearby accommodations; some are helped, some are not.

A far less costly alternative, if only more were available, is a new nontoxic living complex. The first of its kind in the nation, Ecology House opened in August, 1994, in Marin County, California. The two-story, 11-unit apartment building features no wall-to-wall carpets, no fireplaces, draperies, or furnaces. Floors are tiled, paint is nontoxic, and heating is by hot water flowing through metal pipes.

A community room addresses the fundamental desire to visit with friends.

"You can't believe the social isolation that goes with this disease," says one resident, whose disability forced her to quit her job. "Just the idea of being around people like myself, and not having to explain anything or worry about [the scent of] their hair shampoo—is incredible."

Financing for the project came from private and public funds, including a $1.5 million grant from the U.S. Department of Housing and Urban Development, which recognized MCS as a disability in 1993. Would-be tenants were required to provide a doctor's diagnosis of disabling MCS and proof of low income. So many people applied, the "winners" had to be picked by lottery.

The first tenants, however, have reported health problems—a discouraging note. Leaders of the Environmental Health Network, who helped launch Ecology House, do point out that it's very much a pilot project and a learning experience. They still hope to see similar units spring up all over the country.

MEDICAL TREATMENT

Doctors occasionally provide medical therapy for MCS patients. Those who experience an imbalance of *Candida albicans*, a yeast-like flora normally found in the gastrointestinal tract, often develop a mouth infection called thrush, vaginal monilia, or other related problems. These can be successfully treated with an antifungal drug such as nystatin or the newer, faster-acting fluconazole (Diflucan).

Immunologist Alan Levin, M.D., gives many MCS patients injections of "transfer factor," a therapy he helped develop that is not yet widely available.

"I call it immunologic chicken soup," he explains. "It's a mix of various chemical compounds that stimulate the immune system. Other medications may help more but they have more side effects. Transfer factor isn't standardized—every doctor makes his own—and it's not a potent medication. It just gives the patient a nice, subtle boost."

Because MCS is chronic and debilitating, affected persons can lose their jobs, friends, even their mates. Coping with such stresses presents an enormous challenge and frequently leads those who can afford it to seek professional help. Psychotherapy can be invaluable, providing the therapist understands and acknowledges the illness and is sympathetic.

Be sure to question thoroughly any doctor you're considering. Words like "hysteria" and "delusion" should send immediate warning signals.

MCS is a real illness, no matter what opponents argue. The suffering and deprivation that go with it are not imaginary. Battles have been won, scientists have begun to open their minds, and major government agencies now recognize the validity of this diagnosis. But the struggle for compassion continues.

PART VI

HELP YOURSELF TO HEALTH

The human immune system is an army of soldiers—actually, white blood cells—programmed to protect every inch of your body, on 24-hour alert, and trained to fight off any substances perceived as invaders. These can be disease-causing agents such as bacteria and viruses. Or, as you know by now, they can also be harmless substances such as pollens and house dust.

Despite the immune system's imperfections, your body's main line of defense against disease must be kept in prime condition. That means guarding against enemies of the mind as well as the body. Negative emotions such as stress, anxiety, anger, and hostility can take an immense toll on your well-being—far greater, perhaps, than you realize.

That's why it's vital to see your body as a whole: to consider your mental, emotional, and spiritual health, as well as your ability to relax, your willingness to enjoy, even your capacity to love.

CHAPTER 19

NEW AGE THERAPIES

A 1993 study reported in the *New England Journal of Medicine* showed that almost 10 percent of allergy patients have sought relief in one or more types of "unconventional therapy." The study defines this term to mean "commonly used interventions neither taught widely in U.S. medical schools nor generally available in U.S. hospitals."

At one end of the spectrum are such mind-body approaches as biofeedback, stress reduction, hypnosis, relaxation training, and support groups, which more and more doctors are beginning to accept. Acupuncture, chiropractic, and homeopathy fall somewhere in the middle range, and spiritual healing, mental imagery, and herbal medicine still raise eyebrows.

Few responsible scientists believe that the mind can cure cancer or that you can think away allergies and asthma, but research shows that thoughts, beliefs, and emotions can have a major impact on physical health. If you doubt the mind-body connection, look at your own sexuality. Can you deny the link between thought and physical response?

Some physicians feel that straying from the mainstream should be discouraged, that focusing attention on alternative therapies gives credence to quacks, charlatans, and assorted faith healers. Unscrupulous souls do abound to prey on the gullible, but you can protect yourself by watching out for these types:

- Massive egos who plaster their names and pictures all over magazines, billboards, and labels of whatever product(s) they're pushing.

- Pitchmen who bombard the media with scientific-sounding ads based on semi-truths. (If strengthening the lungs helps breathing, the $29.95 packet of balloons is "doctor-proven to aid patients with asthma.")

- Smooth talkers who use charm and persuasion rather than medical data to entice you into buying their product or trying their "therapy."

- Double-talkers who dress up their treatments in "healthspeak." If anyone offers you a "lymphatic drainage massage," a "purifying herbal wrap," or a "detoxifying mineral mud soak," hold onto your wallet. Ingredients in "exfoliating muds" and scrubs can also cause allergic reactions.

- Super salespersons who insist that only they have the cure for your ailment (for example, shark cartilage for cancer) and that medical doctors won't acknowledge this miracle because they make too much money treating the disease.

- Hustlers selling megadoses of anything. Vitamins, Chinese "cleansing" herbs, and mysterious "energy" pills can all have serious side effects.

- Persons who charge exorbitant prices for "rare" or "exotic" ingredients such as mink placenta.

- Anyone who tries to win you over with unsubstantiated letters, claims, or before-and-after photos instead of scientific data.

Quackery notwithstanding, many in the medical profession have bestowed their belated blessings on some ancient healing methods that had been scorned for years.

ACUPUNCTURE

There is no definitive scientific evidence that acupuncture works, yet according to the FDA, about 12 million acupuncture treatments are performed annually in the United States.

There *is* evidence that acupuncture prods nerves in the skin and muscles to signal the brain to release endorphins, morphine-like chemicals that relieve pain and induce a sense of well-being.

Relief of migraines, abdominal cramps, and other allergy-related discomforts might well explain why certain patients believe in acupuncture. Asthma and hay fever also improve in some cases, possibly due to endorphin euphoria, the placebo effect, more relaxed breathing, or other body reactions that remain a mystery.

If you're considering an invasive therapy such as acupuncture for asthma or allergy relief, here's what to do:

1. Check with your doctor. Be sure you've tried appropriate medication before attempting any alternative therapy.

2. Choose your technician with care. Ask if he or she has a license to practice acupuncture. (Twenty-nine states have legalized the practice and require a license.)

3. If your prospective acupuncturist is a physician, make sure he or she belongs to the American Academy of Medical Acupuncture, which requires at least 200 hours of training. Call their referral service at 800-521-2262, or the Academy at 213-937-5514.

4. If your technician is not a physician, check with the National Commission for the Certification of Acupuncturists. They charge $3 for a list of certified nonphysicians. Phone 202-232-1404 for information.

5. If neither of the previous two items apply, inquire if the technician attended a school accredited by the National Council of Schools and Colleges of Acupuncture. Don't choose anyone whose credentials can't be checked.

6. Talk to your insurance company. Some will pay only when a physician does the needling. Currently, no federal programs such as Medicare or Medicaid reimburse for acupuncture.

7. Discuss fees. Nonphysicians charge $30 to $75 for a first visit, less for follow-ups. Physicians may charge more.

8. Discuss treatment. Is it painful? (Most who have tried it say no.) Where are the needles applied? Are they preheated? Twirled? Wired to electric current? How long do they stay in? When can I expect results?

9. Be sure your acupuncturist uses a new set of sterile, disposable needles for each treatment. *Never* agree to reused needles even if they've been sterilized.

10. Know when to stop. If you don't see results after six treatments, if the acupuncturist tells you to change medication or doctors, or if he or she wants to sell you an expensive herbal concoction, *caveat emptor*—let the buyer beware.

BIOFEEDBACK

Born in the 1960s, biofeedback is a technique that teaches you to gain control of some of your involuntary physical responses, such as heart rate, breathing, and blood flow. A trained specialist wires you to a sensitive recording device that feeds back information on immediate body reactions *while they are happening.* The information may come through an image on a screen, flashing lights, a fluctuating needle on a dial, or beeps in your earphones. The instructor then helps you apply this information to change internal body processes.

Biofeedback trainers report very good results with migraine patients, good results with asthmatic children and teenagers, moderate success with asthmatic adults, and less success with adults over 55 who have had asthma for many years. Proponents claim that even if the training doesn't cure all the symptoms, it teaches asthmatics to breathe more easily.

Fees are about $125 for each 45-minute session, usually once a week for six to eight weeks. If your doctor recommends biofeedback, insurance will usually cover it.

The Biofeedback Certification Institute of America, 10200 West 44th Avenue, Suite 304, Wheat Ridge, CO 80033, publishes a directory of practitioners. Send a self-addressed stamped envelope (SASE) to receive a list of names in your area.

CHIROPRACTIC

Traditional chiropractic is a noninvasive, nondrug, nonsurgical therapy. It holds that correcting misalignments of the spine by manual readjustment allows the body to heal itself.

More than 50,000 licensed chiropractors, the third-largest group of health practitioners in the nation (after doctors and dentists), make this specialty somewhat more mainstream and less "alternative."

For the most part, however, chiropractic remains apart from conventional medicine. Along with spine manipulations, many practitioners give valuable nutritional advice, as well as suggestions for proper shoe fit, improved posture, and better sitting and sleeping positions. Others, however, still tout such controversial techniques as herbal medicine, megavitamin therapy, and colonic irrigation that can weaken the intestinal wall and cause digestive problems.

Some asthmatics appear to breathe more easily after treatments, but specific claims that chiropractic can relieve allergy-related headaches, fatigue, weakness, and joint aches are not supported by scientific evidence.

If you're considering chiropractic, check first with your physician. As with all alternative therapies, this should be a supplement to standard medical treatment.

Don't choose a chiropractor from the Yellow Pages or a newspaper ad, and be suspicious of anyone who makes extravagant claims, fails to take a detailed medical history from you, practices psychoanalysis, orders repeated X rays, sells medicines, vitamins, or homeopathic remedies, or wants you to sign a costly long-term contract.

Ask your doctor for names of reputable practitioners or call the National Association for Chiropractic Medicine (NACM) at 713-280-8262 for a referral list.

HERBAL MEDICINE

Plants are the basis for 25 percent of all prescription drugs, so it's not too far-fetched to imagine that thousands of scientifically untested plants might also have medicinal properties.

Proponents of herbalism claim that pharmaceutical companies don't develop more plant medications because it's too risky an investment. Millions of dollars must be spent preparing documents for FDA approval, and plants cannot be patented.

Advocates believe that herbs can treat almost every medical condition imaginable, especially diseases of the blood and the respiratory, nervous, gastrointestinal, and genitourinary systems.

Herbalists prepare remedies in suppository, lotion, ointment, pill, and liquid form—usually a tea that the patient sips several times a day. Both herbalists and physicians warn against brewing your own herbal tea. People have reported severe diarrhea from buckthorn and senna, hallucinations from burdock and jimson weed, and stomach cramps from juniper berries, mistletoe, and nutmeg. Many do-it-yourselfers end up in emergency rooms.

A recent resurgence of interest in herbal medicine has led to stepped-up research all over the world. Millions of Asians, Africans, and Russians use plant remedies in combination with traditional treatment.

Nevertheless, this is not ripe experimental ground for allergic persons. Despite ads for "all-natural" medications such as the Chinese herb ephedra to replace the "manufactured" drug pseudoephedrine, herbs can pose special dangers. Their purity and safety are not regulated by the FDA, and many are full of molds, dust, and bacteria, as well as having toxic properties that can damage the liver.

HOMEOPATHY

Like herbalism, homeopathy is a form of alternative medicine that uses natural substances. Homeopathy, however, seeks to cure illness by using extremely diluted preparations of herbs, minerals, and animal extracts to provoke symptoms resembling the patient's own symptoms. A conventional doctor might treat your runny nose with an antihistamine; a homeopath might have you smell a raw onion to make your nose run more, supposedly flushing the illness out of your system.

The reasoning behind homeopathy, first proposed by German physician Samuel Hahnemann in the late 1700s, is that "like cures like." He believed, as do modern proponents, that while high doses of certain substances intensify the symptoms of disease, minute doses strengthen the body's defense mechanisms and stimulate its "vital force."

One problem allergic patients have is that homeopathic remedies, even those widely advertised and sold in drugstores, don't target the immune system, where allergies start, but seek to harness some mysterious body power.

Most homeopathic remedies are harmless, but they probably won't help you, either. Their danger lies in the risk that you might forego needed medical treatment.

HYPNOSIS

Once thought of as a theatrical gimmick, hypnosis has become a legitimate and effective medical tool. Doctors, dentists, and psychotherapists use it to break bad habits, reduce stress, conquer fears, and cope with pain.

By definition, hypnosis is an induced state of deep relaxation in which the subject is susceptible to suggestions, oblivious to surroundings, and responsive to the instructions of the hypnotist.

Treatment might proceed this way: The hypnotist, speaking in soft, monotonous tones, directs your thoughts to a serene place such as a sunny beach or in front of a warm fire. You're told to focus on that image and remove yourself from your physical reality. The hypnotist then feeds you cues to help you manage the pain of asthma or cope with your allergy, and may suggest certain phrases to repeat to yourself to reinforce the suggestions.

You awake from the trancelike state by opening your eyes and remembering everything that was said. Recall is so vivid, in fact, you may deny you were hypnotized—but if you feel relaxed and mellow, you probably were.

Hypnosis can aid your allergies by helping you to help yourself, especially if you need assistance with such basic disciplines as avoiding chocolate or musty antique shops. Hypnotherapy can also strengthen your will to make overdue changes in your environment and alter some of your negative responses to stress.

Asthmatics may benefit as well. According to a recent British study, hypnotized patients who were told they were being given a bronchodilator showed airway dilation even after taking a placebo.

In general, hypnosis is most effective when you learn self-hypnosis from the therapist and practice it regularly. Treatments range from $40 to $200 an hour, and may or may not be covered by insurance. As with any alternative discipline, don't try it until you've seen your doctor and discussed what you hope to achieve.

Then choose your practitioner carefully. For names of physicians or licensed psychologists who practice hypnotherapy in your area, contact the American Society of Clinical Hypnosis, 2200 East Devon Avenue, Suite 291, Des Plaines, IL 60018, phone 708-297-3317, or send a SASE to The Society for Clinical and Experimental Hypnosis, 128-A Kingspark Drive, Liverpool, NY 13090.

MENTAL IMAGERY

In his book *Meaning and Medicine*, Larry Dossey, M.D., writes of a patient, highly allergic to penicillin, who was given a placebo pill. After he swallowed it he was told, incorrectly, that the pill was not a placebo but penicillin. The man panicked, experienced anaphylaxis, and died.

Why anyone would play such a cruel trick, or why the man couldn't be treated and saved, are mysteries, but the point is well taken. If the mind can be stimulated to turn on a powerful, potentially fatal allergic response, why can't it be stimulated to do the opposite and turn one off?

Proponents of mental imagery, also called visualization, say anything's possible, even reversing the symptoms of cancer. While few mainstream medics would go that far, more and more are beginning to accept this form of autosuggestion as a powerful healing tool.

Visualization has many advantages. It's a nondrug, noninvasive therapy that doesn't call for special equipment or instruction. You can do it anywhere, any time, and at no cost.

Here's how:

- Decide on your goal. Allergy patients can learn to see themselves as healthy, productive persons responsible for their symptoms rather than as helpless victims.

- Follow a relaxation exercise (see Chapter 20). You're much more suggestible when relaxed.

- Close your eyes and create your mental imagery. Try these examples:
  You're strolling down a wooded lane when a gust of wind sends a cloud of pollen wafting toward you. You raise your arm,

snap your fingers, and the pollen turns into a lovely pink (or any color you choose) mist that engulfs you. Its magical healing properties fill you with vitality.

Or: *Imagine yourself lying on warm sand at the beach, listening to the rippling of the waves, smelling the fresh salt water. You breathe deeply, expanding your lungs and allowing the clear ocean air to invigorate you. The oxygen is blue (or any color you choose), and you can see it whooshing through your airways, releasing positive energy as it flows.*

- Finish by picturing yourself achieving your goal.
- Open your eyes and feel alert and refreshed.

Affirmation is another form of mental imagery that seeks to do with word repetition what visualization does with mental pictures.

In his book *Imagery for Healing, Knowledge, and Power*, psychotherapist William Fezler, Ph.D., recalls teaching Sammy, a 9-year-old patient, to work with affirmations, then instructing him via tape:

You can tune out the smell of flowering weeds. You can make your allergy medication expand. The air you breathe smells clear and fresh. The allergy medication you swallow expands infinitely in your bloodstream to vastly heighten its power. You are allergy-free.

"Sammy's first positive results," Dr. Fezler writes, "came from the maximization of his medication."

The boy's mother reported that Sammy responded better to a half-dosage than he had to the full dosage, and within a week, he was back outside playing.

Concludes Dr. Fezler: "The importance of the mind in relation to asthma and allergies was dramatically documented in the now-classic rose-asthma case wherein an allergic patient had a severe attack from a fake rose placed by his side. His believing it was a rose was enough to bring on the allergy, just as you may find that your not believing, not tuning into an allergen, is enough to fend off an attack."

Daily intervals of visualization and/or affirmation will usually bring results within weeks. Practice as often as you can and continue for as long as it seems to help.

PSYCHOTHERAPY

Living with chronic discomfort—whether it's hay fever, asthma, or MCS—isn't easy. Long-term illnesses sap strength, erode confidence and self-esteem, and can engender fear, anger, frustration, and a whole range of negative emotions. Patients often feel the need to seek professional help.

Psychotherapy can take many forms, both mainstream, such as traditional psychoanalysis, and alternative, such as behavior modification, which seeks to change habits by such techniques as conditioning and aversion therapy.

"Asthma can be a very scary experience," says San Francisco psychiatrist Jerome Oremland, M.D., "It's frightening for the patient and for those who observe him. Often it's a real problem for the families. Everything becomes dominated by the person's illness—where to go on vacations so you're not too far from a hospital, how not to upset the person, and so on.

"Asthma patients don't need to learn relaxing so much as they need to identify certain circumstances and let them be. They tend to try to control things that can't be controlled.

"Hay fevers don't seem to be psychosomatically involved," Oremland adds, "but skin eruptions are, especially urticaria or hives. One of my patients—as we talked—her lips swelled and her face became rounder and rounder. She was intensely anxious, and psychotherapy helped her a great deal."

If you're considering psychotherapy, think twice about anyone identified as a "strict Freudian" or who has you lie on a couch. Most modern therapists prefer not to waste your time or money on endless sessions delving into childhood traumas and parental "abuse." They'll talk to you face-to-face, and their treatments are speedier (generally from one to six sessions), less costly, and deal with current problems.

For referrals, call the American Psychiatric Association at 202-682-6000, the American Psychological Association at 202-336-5700; or, for a psychiatric social worker, the National Association of Social Workers, 202-408-8600.

SELF-HELP GROUPS

Before self-help groups existed, people with common problems had little chance to meet each other and share knowledge, experiences, and hope. Today, fortunately, support groups exist for almost every physical illness as well as for a whole range of social, moral, and emotional problems.

These gatherings are generally started by a nonprofessional looking for companionship and support, education, and, in some cases, fellow activists for a cause.

People with MCS, a misunderstood and depressing illness, can benefit greatly from meeting with other MCS patients, sharing what they've learned, and bolstering each other's knowledge that their symptoms are neither imaginary nor unique.

Allergy and asthma patients, particularly the latter, can use self-help groups to compare medical notes and avoidance tips and to help each other cope with some of the lifestyle changes they face.

"I suppose it's a version of misery loves company," says an MCS survivor, "but it's more the feeling that there are others out there who understand your fears and frustrations. A wonderful bond develops when you share like experiences."

To find or form a group, ask your doctor, or contact the American Self-Help Clearinghouse, St. Clares-Riverside Medical Center, 25 Pocono Road, Denville, NJ 07834. The phone number is 201-625-7101 or 201-625-9565.

CHAPTER 20

STRESS-BUSTING

When the demands of your life are greater than the resources you have to deal with them, you become
stressed—overloaded with tension. External events don't cause
the stress; the stress comes in how you perceive and cope with
the problems.

Some stress can be beneficial. Without it, you would never
be able to make love, weep for joy, or feel your heart race with
excitement. Too much stress, however, can be disastrous for allergic persons, triggering hay fever and asthma attacks, increasing susceptibility to allergens and irritants, and leading to major
ailments such as heart disease.

Nevertheless, illness is not the unavoidable price of modern
life. Once you learn to deal with situations, you can prevent
building up so much stress that your "barrel" spills over. Try
these suggestions:

1. Identify the stressors. Ask yourself exactly what's bothering
   you instead of stifling or ignoring your feelings.

2. Look for a solution. Can you change or improve matters,
   and if not, can you accept the problem for now, until such
   time as you can change it?

3. Acceptance means talking to yourself, saying, "Someday I'll
   look back on this and laugh," or "What a wonderful learning experience!" You can't help but learn from what you're

going through, and if the problem arises again, you'll be better equipped to handle it.

4. Reach out to someone you love and trust. A family member or a close friend may offer new perspective. No one can know your feelings or offer to help unless you express yourself. Ventilate your emotions before they build up.

5. If you feel the problem is insurmountable or that you can't handle it alone, consider seeking professional help. A psychotherapist, psychiatric social worker, or mental health counselor can help guide you back to equanimity.

6. Don't be overly self-critical. Sometimes it *is* the other person's fault, and in that case, tell yourself, "That's his/her problem."

7. Think positive thoughts. Tell yourself you're in control. Recount the blessings in your life, the crises you've survived, the physical and emotional resources you have to help you meet the challenge.

8. Daydream. Focus on your next vacation, a compliment you loved, an event you're anticipating. Set goals and imagine achieving them.

9. Pamper yourself. Eat well, sleep well, make time for pleasurable activities. Take laughter breaks with friends, browse in your favorite shops, choose spare-time activities you've always wanted to do. Visit museums, learn calligraphy, buy a home computer, whatever.

10. Build your stamina with exercise. Walking is a terrific way to relax, particularly near a lake or the ocean. Avoid competitive sports and don't force yourself to do strenuous exercises or aerobics unless you enjoy them.

11. At work, learn to say no. When asked to take on an extra task, start with a positive, "I'd love to help you, but. . . ." If possible, end on a positive note. "Try me in a few days, maybe I won't be under so much pressure." Be brief. The longer you talk to a co-worker, the more likely you are to give in.

12. At home, recognize the need for solitude and make time to collect yourself and your thoughts. Family members should understand if you say, "I'm really feeling uptight right now and I need a few minutes alone to unwind."

13. Establish a routine for household chores and delegate responsibility rather than trying to do everything yourself. Arrange for help if you can, and use the time to read a good mystery, see a movie, or listen to music.

14. Plan for emergencies, disasters, and unexpected crises such as locking yourself out of the house. For example, if you're concerned about home security, buy a burglar alarm. Knowing you're protected will give you an added sense of calm and security.

15. Make lists. Tried but true, this old-fashioned stress-buster works. Writing down what you have to do helps you organize, prioritize, and accomplish your chores. Scratch off the items one by one as you do them.

The important point is to take an active role in reducing stress. Don't just let it happen. Untreated or ignored, stress can aggravate any weakness or physical susceptibility you have.

CHRONIC FATIGUE SYNDROME

Sometimes called the Yuppie Disease because it tends to affect overstressed young professionals striving too hard to get ahead, chronic fatigue syndrome (CFS) is not a single ailment, but a complex of symptoms with no obvious cause. Also called chronic fatigue and immune dysfunction syndrome (CFIDS), chronic Epstein-Barr virus (CEBV), and M.E. (myalgic encephalomyelitis), the main characteristic of CFS is fatigue so devastating you can hardly lift your head (some patients have to be carried to the bathroom) and so debilitating that it reduces daily activity by 50 percent for at least six months.

In her book *The Whole Way to Allergy Relief and Prevention*, Jacqueline Krohn, M.D., quotes medical sources who implicate allergy in the baffling syndrome, stating that 75 percent of CFS patients have inhalant, food, drug, or chemical allergies.

There is no lab test for CFS. To make a diagnosis, a doctor must first rule out other possible conditions such as cancer or a major disease, viral infection, mental illness, drug or medication side effects.

The physician must then confirm at least 10 of the following symptoms:

- Anxiety
- Arthralgia (pain in a joint) without swelling or redness
- . Confusion
- Depression and/or suicidal feelings
- Forgetfulness
- Hair loss
- Headaches of a new type or pattern
- Low-grade fever
- Inability to concentrate; difficulty thinking
- Intolerance of alcohol
- Irritability
- Joint pain
- Muscle discomfort or myalgia (pain or aching)
- Muscle weakness
- Night chills
- Numbness
- Prickling sensations or extreme nerve sensitivity
- Shortness of breath
- Sleep disturbance (hypersomnia or insomnia)
- Sore throat
- Swollen or tender lymph nodes
- Visual disturbances (spots, photophobia, blurring)

There's no specific cure for CFS, but early diagnosis, treatment, and emotional support can be effective. Avoidance of allergens, very low doses of antidepressant drugs, aspirin, saltwater gargles, lifestyle changes, stress reduction and relaxation disciplines, regular minimal exercise, bed rest, and healthy eating all help boost spirits as well as body. Some patients benefit from psychological counseling and/or joining a self-help group.

CFS has been reported in all age and economic levels but strikes twice as many women as men, mostly in the 20–45 age group. Some evidence suggests that certain types of CFS may be the result of parasite infections picked up in foreign countries.

Contrary to what many people think, CFS is a valid illness, recognized by mainstream medicine as well as the federal government. If you feel you might have this frustrating ailment, don't accept the condition as permanent or incurable. It doesn't have to be either. Call the Chronic Fatigue and Immune Dysfunction Syndrome (CFIDS) Association of America at 800-442-3437 for an information kit.

THE ART OF RELAXATION

Perhaps the most effective way to reduce stress is to learn how to relax, a skill that can benefit everyone, including CFS patients. Overwhelming evidence indicates that relaxation enhances immune function. How you achieve a relaxed state doesn't really matter as long as you do so.

Hundreds of relaxation techniques from autosuggestion to yoga have come into vogue in recent years. One of the best known is the Hindu practice of transcendental meditation or TM. Neither a philosophy nor a religion, TM requires no beliefs, no faith, no change of lifestyle. It seeks to achieve its calming effect by having you silently repeat a sound, or mantra, while you shut out worldly thoughts.

The TM organization charges $400 to $1,000 for an eight-hour course (spread out over four days) that teaches you how to use your mantra. You may prefer to spend $9.98 on a meditation tape, available in most bookstores, and try to achieve the same results on your own.

Harvard Medical School professor Herbert Benson, M.D., developed a popular Western form of meditation he calls the relaxation response, a somewhat simpler system to reduce stress and produce physiological benefits.

Many meditation techniques begin with progressive muscle relaxation, an exercise to free the body of physical tensions that might distract the mind.

Here's one version:

- Find a quiet spot, loosen your clothing, and sit in a comfortable chair with your feet flat on the floor, your hands resting on your lap. Breathe deeply through your nose, holding the air for several seconds, then exhale. As you exhale, feel the tension flow out of you.

- Start from the toes of your left foot, then your right. Focus on each body part, first tightening, then feeling the tightness melt as you exhale. Work up to your ankles, calves, knees, thighs. Tighten, then release. Continue up through your buttocks, back, shoulders, hands. Relax your forearms, upper arms, neck. Let your jaw go loose and your eyelids float down over your eyes. Allow the wave of relaxation to sweep over your entire body.

- Take a minute to relish the feeling. The key to successful relaxation, according to author/oncologist Ernest H. Rosenbaum, M.D., is to keep the exercise simple and pleasurable. "If the process isn't enjoyable," he says, "chances are it won't be effective. Once it becomes a chore, it will do just what you don't want it to do—*increase* tension."

- Now focus on a single word, phrase, or thought.

- Still breathing deeply and slowly, repeat the word or phrase mentally, concentrate on it, and try to tune out all other thoughts. When your mind wanders, ease it gently back.

- Do this for 5–30 minutes at least once a day, more often when you feel stressed. Set aside a specific time to relax and center yourself, focusing on the positives in your life.

You may want to read some of these suggestions into a tape recorder so you can play them back to yourself later. Tell your doctor what you're doing as this may affect your condition and whatever medication you're taking.

Remember that stress starts in the brain. When you're faced with a difficult time in your life, specific action can help protect your health. The more you're able to relax, neutralize your anxieties, and bolster your immune system, the greater your resistance to all physical ills, including allergy.

Albert Schweitzer once said, "Each patient carries his own doctor inside of him." Mobilizing that inner force can add new dimension to the task of getting well.

EPILOGUE

The troubling news that more people are suffering allergies than ever before translates into the good news that research in this field is at an all-time peak. According to the *Journal of the American Medical Association*, "The specialty of allergy-clinical immunology thrives and we can expect exciting and clinically-useful developments [before the year 2000]."

In IgE-mediated disease, for instance, studies using genetically altered allergens show promise of leading to safer, more effective, easier-to-administer immunotherapy.

Interaction among physicians and scientists at the National Jewish Center for Immunology and Respiratory Medicine is leading to the development of new treatments that emphasize self-management of asthma, as well as new medication to replace oral corticosteroids. Several recent studies linking persistent asthma with low-level viral infection raise the possibility of an antiviral approach to controlling asthma.

A fast-acting nasal spray containing the drug DHE (dihydroergotamine) should be on the market as you read this, and has shown excellent results in treating allergic and nonallergic migraines. Further down the road may be a capsicum nasal spray using capsaicin, the "hot" substance in hot peppers. Now being tested at Johns Hopkins Medical School, the spray appears to have some success in shutting off nasal discharge.

Advances in education and research also offer hope for those with chemical sensitivities. More and more is being learned about reactions to toxic chemicals, electromagnetic fields, fluorescent lights, office machine vapors, and building- and home-related illnesses. New alternatives are constantly being offered to replace household solvents, pesticides and other pollutants, and increasing numbers of intelligent, open-minded persons are recognizing MCS as a real disease, not hysteria.

All in all, there's every reason for optimism. The day will eventually come when scientists unlock the key to the biological mystery known as allergy, and bequeath to history the pains and illnesses that have plagued so many for so long.

NATIONAL ALLERGY AND ASTHMA ORGANIZATIONS

Most will provide written material and information. (See also Appendices B and C.)

ALLERGY AND ASTHMA NETWORK/
    MOTHERS OF ASTHMATICS, INC.
3554 Chain Bridge Rd., Suite 200
Fairfax, VA 22030-2709
800-878-4403 or 703-385-4403

AMERICAN ACADEMY OF ALLERGY
    AND IMMUNOLOGY
611 E. Wells St.
Milwaukee, WI 53202
800-822-ASMA or 414-272-6071
Fax 414-276-3349

AMERICAN ACADEMY OF
    OTOLARYNGIC ALLERGY
1101 Vermont Ave. NW, Suite 302
Washington, DC 20005
202-682-0456

AMERICAN ACADEMY OF
    OTOLARYNGIC ALLERGY—
    HEAD AND NECK SURGERY
One Prince St.
Alexandria, VA 22314
703-836-4444

AMERICAN ALLERGY ASSOCIATION
PO Box 7273
Menlo Park, CA 94026
415-322-1663

AMERICAN BOARD OF ALLERGY
    AND IMMUNOLOGY
215-349-9466

AMERICAN COLLEGE OF ALLERGY
AND IMMUNOLOGY
800 E. Northwest Highway,
Suite 1080
Palatine, IL 60067
800-842-7777 or 708-359-2800

AMERICAN COLLEGE OF CHEST
PHYSICIANS
3300 Dundee Rd.
Northbrook, IL 60062-2340
708-498-1400

AMERICAN IN VITRO ALLERGY AND
IMMUNOLOGY SOCIETY
201-816-1289

AMERICAN LUNG ASSOCIATION
GPO Box 596
New York, NY 10116-0596
800-LUNG-USA, 800-556-6650, or
212-315-8700

ASTHMA AND ALLERGY
FOUNDATION OF AMERICA
(AAFA)
1125 15th St. NW, Suite 502
Washington, DC 20005
800-7-ASTHMA or 202-466-7643

ASTHMA INFORMATION CENTER
PO Box 790
Springhouse, PA 19477-0790
800-727-5400

ASTHMATIC CHILDREN'S
FOUNDATION
PO Box 568
Spring Valley Rd.
Ossining, NY 10562
914-762-2110

ECZEMA ASSOCIATION
1221 SW Yamhill, Suite 303
Portland, OR 97205
503-228-4430

FOOD ALLERGY NETWORK
4744 Holly Ave.
Fairfax, VA 22030-5647
800-929-4040 or 703-691-3179
Fax 703-691-2713

FOUNDATION FOR ALLERGY CARE
AND TREATMENT (FACT)
301-588-1802

NATIONAL ASTHMA EDUCATION
PROGRAM INFORMATION CENTER
(NAEPP)
PO Box 30105
Bethesda, MD 20824-0105
301-251-1223

NATIONAL FOUNDATION FOR
ASTHMA, INC.
PO Box 30069
Tucson, AZ 85751-0069
602-323-6046

NATIONAL HEART, LUNG AND
BLOOD INSTITUTE INFORMATION
CENTER
PO Box 30105
Bethesda, MD 20824-0105
301-251-1222

NATIONAL INSTITUTE OF ALLERGY
AND INFECTIOUS DISEASES
(NIAID)
Clinical Center Communications
9000 Rockville Pike
Building 10, Room 1C255
Bethesda, MD 20892
301-496-2563

NATIONAL JEWISH CENTER FOR
IMMUNOLOGY AND RESPIRATORY
MEDICINE
1400 Jackson St.
Denver, CO 80206
800-222-LUNG, 800-552-LUNG
(for info), or 303-388-4461

PARENTS OF ASTHMATIC/ALLERGIC
CHILDREN
1412 Marathon Drive
Fort Collins, CO 80524
303-842-7395

ENVIRONMENTAL HEALTH RESOURCES

NATIONAL ORGANIZATIONS

(See also Appendices A and C.)

AMERICAN ACADEMY OF
ENVIRONMENTAL MEDICINE
PO Box 16106
Denver, CO 80216
303-622-9755
(Will send names of doctors in
your area sensitive to MCS)

CHEMICAL INJURY INFORMATION
NETWORK (CIIN)
PO Box 301
White Sulphur Springs, MT 59645
406-547-2255
(Newsletter: *Our Toxic Times*)

ENVIRONMENTAL ACCESS RESEARCH
NETWORK (EARN)
Route 1, Box 16-6
Epping, ND 58843
701-859-6367

ENVIRONMENTAL HEALTH
NETWORK
PO Box 1155
Larkspur, CA 94977
415-541-5075
(Bimonthly newsletter: *The New
Reactor*)

HUMAN ECOLOGY ACTION
LEAGUE, INC. (HEAL)
PO Box 49126
Atlanta, GA 30359-1126
404-248-1898
(Quarterly magazine: *The Human
Ecologist*)

INFORMED CONSENT
PO Box 1984
Williston, ND 58802
(Bimonthly magazine)

MCS REFERRAL AND RESOURCES
2326 Pickwick Rd.
Baltimore, MD 21207-6631
410-448-3319
Fax 410-448-3317

NATIONAL CENTER FOR
 ENVIRONMENTAL HEALTH
 STRATEGIES (NCEHS)
1100 Rural Ave.
Voorhees, NJ 08043
609-429-5358
(Newsletter: *The Delicate Balance*;
 membership includes referral
 network of medical, legal, and
 environmental health specialists who have experience with
 MCS)

PRICE-POTTENGER NUTRITION
 FOUNDATION (MCS Resource
 Center)
PO Box 2614
La Mesa, CA 91943-2614
800-366-3748 or 619-574-7763
Fax 619-574-1314

OTHER INFORMATION RESOURCES

(See also Appendices A and B.)

ACUPUNCTURE: AMERICAN
  ACADEMY OF MEDICAL
  ACUPUNCTURE
800-521-2262 or 213-937-5514

ACUPUNCTURE: NATIONAL
  COMMISSION FOR THE
  CERTIFICATION OF
  ACUPUNCTURISTS
202-232-1404

ALLERGY HOTLINE (organic foods
  newsletter)
PO Box 161132
Altamonte Springs, FL 32716-
  1132
407-628-1377

ALLERGY INFORMATION
  ASSOCIATION
65 Tromley Drive, Suite 10
Etobicoke, Ontario M9B5Y7
Canada

ALLERGY PUBLICATIONS
PO Box 640
Menlo Park, CA 94026

AMERICAN BOARD OF MEDICAL
  SPECIALTIES
800-733-2267 or 800-776-CERT
(to verify certification status of
  physician)

AMERICAN SELF-HELP
CLEARINGHOUSE (for help in
finding or forming support
group)
St. Clares-Riverside Medical
Center
25 Pocono Rd.
Denville, NJ 07834
201-625-7101 or 201-625-9565
Fax 201-625-8848

BETTER BREATHERS CLUB
800-556-6650

BIOFEEDBACK CERTIFICATION
INSTITUTE OF AMERICA
10200 W. 44th Ave., Suite 304
Wheat Ridge, CO 80033
303-420-2902

BUILDING OWNERS AND MANAGERS
ASSOCIATION INTERNATIONAL
(info about healthy buildings)
PO Box 79330
Baltimore, MD 21279-0330
800-426-6292

CARPET AND RUG INSTITUTE
(info on carpet emissions)
800-882-8846

CELIAC SPRUE
For info, call NIDDK,
NIH: 301-496-3583

CENTER FOR ENVIRONMENTAL
MEDICINE (detox clinic)
7510 Northforest Drive
N. Charleston, SC 29418
803-572-1600

CENTERS FOR DISEASE CONTROL
AND PREVENTION
4770 Buford Highway NE
Atlanta, GA 30341-3724
800-488-7330

CHEMICAL INJURY RESEARCH
FOUNDATION (CIRF)
3639 N. Pearl St.
Tacoma, WA 98407
206-752-6677
Fax 206-752-0735

CHIROPRACTIC: NATIONAL
ASSOCIATION FOR CHIROPRACTIC
MEDICINE (NACM)
713-280-8262

CHRONIC FATIGUE AND IMMUNE
DYSFUNCTION SYNDROME
(CFIDS) ASSOCIATION OF
AMERICA
PO Box 220398
Charlotte, NC 28222-0398
800-442-3437 or 900-896-2343
(pay-per-call info line)
Fax 704-365-9755

COMPLETE DRUG REFERENCE
Box 10637
Des Moines, IA 50336
515-237-4903

COMPUTER-RELATED HEALTH ISSUES:
Apple: 800-776-2333
IBM: 800-772-2227

SAFE TECHNOLOGIES CORP.:
800-638-9121

DISABILITY RESOURCE CENTER OF
TUCSON
800-234-0344 or 602-624-6452

ENERGY EFFICIENCY AND
RENEWABLE ENERGY
CLEARINGHOUSE (EREC)
PO Box 3048
Merrifield, VA 22116
800-DOE-EREC

ENVIRONMENTAL HEALTH CENTER
(detox clinic)
8345 Walnut Hill Lane, Suite 205
Dallas, TX 75231
214-368-4132

ENVIRONMENTAL HEALTH
COALITION (pesticide
alternatives)
PO Box 8426
San Diego, CA 92102
619-235-0281

ENVIRONMENTAL HEALTH LETTER
PO Box 3638
Syracuse, NY 13220
315-455-7862

ENVIRONMENTAL RESEARCH
FOUNDATION (info on
hazardous waste)
PO Box 5036
Annapolis, MD 21403-7036
410-263-1584

FOOD AND DRUG ADMINISTRATION
(FDA)
Center for Food Safety and
Applied Nutrition, Division of
Colors and Cosmetics
200 C St. SW
Washington, D.C. 20204
800-FDA-4010 or 202-245-1317

FOOD AND NUTRITION
INFORMATION CENTER (for info
about nutrition resources)
National Agricultural Library,
Room 304
Beltsville, MD 20705
301-344-3719

FORMALDEHYDE INSTITUTE INC.
1330 Connecticut Ave. NW
Washington, D.C. 20036

GULF WAR SYNDROME
California Association of Persian
Gulf Veterans
PO Box 3661
Santa Cruz, CA 95063
408-476-6684

GULF WAR SYNDROME
Desert Storm Veterans Coalition
800-307-1330

GULF WAR SYNDROME
Major Richard Haines, U.S. Army
Reserve
4247 Valley Terrace
New Albany, IN 47150
812-948-9366

HEALTHY HOUSE INSTITUTE
7471 N. Shiloh Rd.
Unionville, IN 47468
812-332-5073

HUD'S FAIR HOUSING ACT INFO
800-795-7915

HUMAN ECOLOGY FOUNDATION
OF CANADA
46 Highway #8
Dundas, Ontario L9H4V3
Canada
414-628-8241

HYPNOSIS: AMERICAN SOCIETY
OF CLINICAL HYPNOSIS
2200 E. Devon Ave., Suite 291
Des Plaines, IL 60018
708-297-3317

HYPNOSIS: SOCIETY FOR CLINICAL
AND EXPERIMENTAL HYPNOSIS
128-A Kingspark Drive
Liverpool, NY 13090

INDOOR AIR QUALITY INFORMATION
CLEARING HOUSE (IAQ Info)
Environmental Protection
Agency
PO Box 37133
Washington, D.C. 20013-7133
800-438-4318 or 301-585-9020
Fax 301-588-3408

LABOR OCCUPATIONAL HEALTH
PROGRAM (computer-related
issues)
University of California School of
Public Health
2515 Channing Way
Berkeley, CA 94720
510-642-5507

MAST IMMUNOSYSTEMS TECHNICAL
SERVICE (for blood test)
630 Clyde Court
Mountain View, CA 94043
800-233-6273

MEDIC ALERT (for medical ID)
2323 Colorado Ave.
Turlock, CA 95382
800-432-5378

MED-DATA INFORMATION SERVICES
(for medical ID)
PO Box 150031
Cape Coral, FL 33915

NATIONAL ACADEMY OF SCIENCES
INSTITUTE OF MEDICINE
(environmental medicine and
medical school)
2101 Constitution Ave. NW
Washington, D.C. 20418
202-334-1716

NATIONAL DIGESTIVE DISEASES
INFORMATION CLEARINGHOUSE
(for educational materials on
lactose intolerance)
301-468-6344

NATIONAL INSTITUTE FOR
OCCUPATIONAL SAFETY AND
HEALTH (NIOSH) (to request
health hazard evaluation)
Mailstop R-11
4676 Columbia Parkway
Cincinnati, OH 45226
800-356-4674

NATIONAL PESTICIDE
TELECOMMUNICATIONS
NETWORK (EPA)
800-858-PEST
In Texas: 806-743-3091

NATIONAL SANITATION
FOUNDATION (info on water
filters)
PO Box 130140-PVN
Ann Arbor, MI 48113-0140

NORTHEAST CENTER FOR
ENVIRONMENTAL MEDICINE (to
identify molds, formaldehyde
in your home)
2800 W. Genesee St.
Syracuse, NY 13219
315-488-2856
Fax 315-488-7518

OCCUPATIONAL HEALTH AND 3M
SAFETY PRODUCTS DIVISION
(formaldehyde test kit)
220-7W 3M Center
St. Paul, MN 55144-1000
800-388-3458 or 612-733-8029

OCCUPATIONAL SAFETY AND
HEALTH ADMINISTRATION
(OSHA)
Office of Information and
Consumer Affairs,
Room N-3647
200 Constitution Ave. NW
Washington, D.C. 20210
202-219-8151

PAN AMERICAN ALLERGY SOCIETY
(for physician referrals)
PO Box 947
Fredericksburg, TX 78624
512-997-7467

PSYCHOTHERAPY: AMERICAN
PSYCHIATRIC ASSOCIATION
202-682-6000

PSYCHOTHERAPY: AMERICAN
PSYCHOLOGICAL ASSOCIATION
202-336-5700

PSYCHOTHERAPY: NATIONAL
ASSOCIATION OF SOCIAL
WORKERS
202-408-8600

QUESTIONABLE DOCTORS
($15 for state list)
Public Citizen
Publications Dept. PL0394
2000 P St. NW, Suite 600
Washington, D.C., 20036
202-833-3000

RADON HOTLINE (operated by the National Safety Council, EPA)
800-SOS-RADON for info kit
800-55-RADON for questions

SAFE BUILDINGS ALLIANCE
Metropolitan Square
655 15th St. NW, Suite 1200
Washington, DC 20005
202-879-5120

SAFE DRINKING WATER HOTLINE
202-382-5533

SOCIETY FOR THE STUDY OF
BIOCHEMICAL INTOLERANCE
1675 N. Freedom Blvd., Suite 11E
Provo, UT 84606
801-373-8500

SOYFOODS ASSOCIATION OF
AMERICA
415-393-9697

TOXIC CARPET INFORMATION
EXCHANGE
PO Box 39344
Cincinnati, OH 45239

TOXIC SUBSTANCE CONTROL ACT
ASSISTANCE INFORMATION
SERVICE (EPA)
202-554-1404

U.S. BORAX
Public Relations
26877 Tourney Rd.
Valencia, CA 91355
800-457-8739

U.S. CONSUMER PRODUCT SAFETY
COMMISSION (complaints about products)
Washington, DC 20207
800-638-CPSC

U.S. DEPARTMENT OF AGRICULTURE
(nutrition info)
800-535-4555

WOLVERTON ENVIRONMENTAL
SERVICES
1105 Highway 43 East
Picayune, MS 39466
601-799-3807

WHERE TO SEND FOR PRODUCTS

Most of these companies offer free catalogs of products for allergen-sensitive persons. (This list does not represent an endorsement of any company or its merchandise.)

HOME PRODUCTS

ABSOLUTE ENVIRONMENTALS
ALLERGY STORE
2615 S. University Drive
Davie, FL 33328
800-771-2246 or 305-472-0128
Fax 305-474-0133

ALLENS NATURALLY
PO Box 339, Dept. H
Farmington, MI 48332-0339
800-352-8971

ALLERGY ALTERNATIVES
440 Godfrey Drive
Windsor, CA 95492
800-838-1514

ALLERGY ASTHMA
TECHNOLOGY LTD.
PO Box 18398
Chicago, IL 60618
800-621-5545
Fax 312-465-7619

ALLERGY CLEAN ENVIRONMENTS
501 Station Ave.
Haddon Heights, NJ 08035
800-882-4110
Fax 609-546-1466

ALLERGY CONTROL PRODUCTS
96 Danbury Rd., PO Box 793
Ridgefield, CT 06877
800-422-DUST

ALLERGY PUBLICATIONS
PO Box 640
Menlo Park, CA 94026

ALLERGY SUPPLY COMPANY
11994 Star Court
Herndon, VA 22071
800-323-6744

AMERICAN ENVIRONMENTAL
    HEALTH FOUNDATION
8345 Walnut Hill Lane, Suite 225
Dallas, TX 75231
800-428-2343 or 214-361-9515
Fax 214-691-8432

AUTO-TECH LIMITED
PO Box 777
Rancho Cordova, CA 95441
916-488-0668
Fax 916-863-7884

BIO-INTEGRAL RESOURCE CENTER
    (BIRC) (pest management)
PO Box 7414
Berkeley, CA 94707
510-524-2567
Fax 510-524-1758

CARING FOR YOU
1139 Cotswald Court
Sunnyvale, CA 94087
408-296-7968

CHARCOAL MASKS
Sandra DenBraber, RN
114 Ray St.
Arlington, TX 76010
817-469-9626

COASTLINE PRODUCTS
PO Box 6397
Santa Ana, CA 92706
800-554-4111 or -4112
Fax 800-554-6861

COTTON PLACE
PO Box 59721H
Dallas, TX 75229
214-243-4149

COTTONTAILS ORGANIC-WEAR
3684 Hicks Hill Rd.
Friendship, NY 14739
716-973-3000

DONA DESIGNS (organic bedding)
1611 Bent Tree St.
Seagoville, TX 75159

EHS (Environmental Health
    Safety) PRODUCTS, INC.
3500 W. 75th St.
Prairie Village, KS 66208
800-430-5129

ENGEN DRUG ALLERGY DIVISION
    (allergy relief products)
PO Box 218
Karlstad, MN 56732
800-648-0074 or 218-436-2485

ENVIRO-CLEAN
30 Walnut Ave.
Floral Park, NY 11001-9866
800-466-1425 or 516-775-1425

ENVIRONMENTAL OUTFITTERS
44 Crosby St.
New York, NY 10012
800-238-5008 or 212-334-9659
Fax 212-226-8084

ENVIRONMENTAL
    PURIFICATION SYSTEMS
PO Box 191
Concord, CA 94522
415-682-7231

GARNET HILL
262 Main St.
Franconia, NH 03580-0262
800-622-6216
Fax 603-823-9578

HEALTH CENTER FOR BETTER
    LIVING, INC.
6189 Taylor Rd.
Naples, FL 33942-1865
813-566-2611
Fax 813-566-9508

JANICE CORPORATION (skin and
    allergy products)
198 U.S. Highway 46
Budd Lake, NJ 07828-3001
800-JANICES or 201-691-2979

LIFESTYLE RESOURCE
Dept. BBKK03
4184 Taylor Rd.
Batavia, OH 45103
800-872-5200

LIVING SOURCE
7005 Woodway Drive, Suite 214
Waco, TX 76712
800-662-8787 or 817-776-4878
Fax 817-776-9329

MOTHER HART'S NATURAL
    PRODUCTS FOR HOME & BODY
PO Box 4229, Dept. PV
Boynton Beach, FL 33424-4929
407-738-5866 or 407-738-0732

NATIONAL ALLERGY SUPPLY, INC.
4400 Georgia Highway 120
PO Box 1658
Duluth, GA 30136
800-522-1448
Fax 404-623-5568

NATURAL ANIMAL, INC.
    (pet products)
PO Box 1177
St. Augustine, FL 32085
800-274-7387

N.E.E.D.S. (National Ecological &
    Environmental Delivery
    Systems)
527 Charles Ave. 12-A
Syracuse, NY 13209
800-634-1380
Fax 800-295-NEED

NIGRA ENTERPRISES
    (purification products)
5699 Kanan Rd.
Agoura, CA 91301
818-889-6877

NILFISK OF AMERICA
    (vacuum cleaners)
300 Technology Drive
Malvern, PA 19355
800-241-9420

RADIANT HEATER CORP.
PO Box 60
74100-2 W. Front St.
Greenport, NY 11944
800-331-6408

REAL GOODS
966 Mazzoni St.
Ukiah, CA 95482-3471
800-762-7325
Fax 707-468-9486

REFLECTIONS (organic clothing)
Route 2, Box 24P40
Dept. HL 994
Trinity, TX 75862
409-594-9019
Fax 409-594-5196

ROMAN RESEARCH, INC. (earrings
    for nickel-sensitive persons)
33 Riverside Drive
Pembroke, MA 02359-1910
800-451-5700

SAFE READING AND COMPUTER
    BOX CO.
1158 N. Huron
Linwood, MI 48634
517-697-3989

SELF CARE CATALOG
5850 Shellmound St., Suite 390
Emeryville, CA 94662-0813
800-345-3371

FOODS

ALLERGY RESOURCES
PO Box 888
Palmer Lake, CO 80133
800-USE-FLAX

ALL OF WASHINGTON'S BEST
16528 NE 35th Court
Suite QQ103
Redmond, WA 98052
800-840-SAFE
Fax 206-727-6801

OMEGA NUTRITION
6505 Aldrich Rd.
Bellingham, WA 98226
800-661-3529

ORGANIC FOODWORKS
Box A-1, RR #3
Howard, PA 16841
814-355-9850 or 604-322-8862
Fax 604-327-2932

PAMELA'S PRODUCTS INC.
156 Utah Ave.
S. San Francisco, CA 94080
415-952-4546

FOOD FAMILIES

If you're allergic to a food in one botanical family, you may be sensitive to other foods in the same family. This is called cross-reactivity.

Here are some popular foods and their relatives:

Almond—Apricot, cherry, nectarine, peach, plum, prune

Apple—Crabapple, pear, pectin, quince, rosehips

Asparagus—Chive, garlic, leek, onion, shallot

Avocado—Bay leaf, cinnamon

Banana—Arrowroot, plantain

Basil—Marjoram, mint, oregano, peppermint, rosemary, sage, savory, spearmint, thyme

Beef—Buffalo, butter, cheese, gelatin, goat, lamb, milk, pork, sheep, veal, and all related products

Beet—Beet sugar, chard, spinach

Black pepper—White pepper

Blueberry—Cranberry, huckleberry

Buckwheat—Rhubarb, sorrel

Cabbage—Bok choy, broccoli, Brussels sprouts, cauliflower, Chinese cabbage, collards, horseradish, kale, kohlrabi, mustard, radish, rutabaga, turnip, watercress

Carrot—Anise, caraway, celeriac, celery, coriander, cumin, dill, fennel, papaya, parsley, parsnip

Cashew—Mango, pistachio

Cheese (hard)—Mushrooms, truffles, yeast

Chicken—Cornish hen, duck, pheasant, quail, turkey, and all their eggs

Clove—Allspice, guava

Cocoa—Chocolate, cocoa butter, cola

Coconut—Date, hearts of palm

Codfish—Haddock, pollack, whiting

Cottonseed oil—Okra

Crab—Crayfish, lobster, prawn, shrimp

Currant—Gooseberry

Deer—Elk, moose, reindeer

Gin—Pine nut

Ginger—Cardamom, curry, turmeric

Grape—Brandy, champagne, cream of tartar, raisin, wine, wine vinegar

Lettuce—Artichoke, chamomile, chicory, dandelion, endive, escarole, tarragon, safflower, sesame, sunflower seed, and their oils

Melon—Cantaloupe, casaba, chayote, cucumber, gherkin, honeydew, pumpkin, squash, watermelon

Nutmeg—Mace

Olive —Olive oil

Orange—Grapefruit, kumquat, lemon, lime, tangerine

Oyster—Abalone, clam, mussel, scallop, snail, squid

Peanut—Alfalfa, bean (garbanzo, kidney, lima, navy, pinto, soy, string), bean sprouts, black-eyed pea, carob, guar gum, hydrolyzed vegetable protein, lentil, licorice, pea

Pomegranate—Grenadine

Potato—Pepper (cayenne, chili, red, green), eggplant, paprika, pimiento, tobacco, tomato

Salmon—Trout

Sea bass—Grouper

Sole—Flounder, halibut, plaice, turbot

Sweet potato—Jicama, yam

Tuna—Albacore, bonito, mackerel

Walnut—Butternut, hickory nut, pecan

Wheat—Bamboo shoots, barley, corn, graham flour, millet, molasses, oat, rice, rye, sorghum, sugarcane, wild rice

GLOSSARY

ABSORPTION   The process by which food substances are taken in through the intestinal wall and passed into the bloodstream.

ACARACIDE   Mite-killing product.

ACUPRESSURE   The Chinese technique of massaging or putting pressure on specific body points to relieve pain.

ACUPUNCTURE   The Chinese technique of puncturing specific body points with needles to relieve pain or disease symptoms.

ACUTE   Extremely sharp or severe, as in pain; refers to a sudden intense illness or reaction.

ADDITIVES   Substances such as preservatives or coloring agents added to foods to enhance appearance, taste, or freshness.

ADRENAL GLANDS   A pair of glands, one located above each kidney. The outer core produces cortisone; the inner core or medulla produces adrenaline.

ADRENALINE   A hormone secreted by the inner core of the

adrenal glands. Trademark name: Adrenalin. (See *epineph-rine.*)

AFFIRMATION   The act of making a positive statement and re-peating it over and over to enhance healing.

AIRWAYS   The air passages from nose to lungs.

ALLERGEN   Any substance that causes an allergic reaction; an antigen, usually a protein of high molecular weight.

ALLERGENIC   Causing or producing an allergic reaction.

ALLERGIC RHINITIS   Hay fever; seasonal or perennial nasal in-flammation due to allergy.

ALLERGY   A hypersensitivity to a specific substance that will not produce a reaction in nonallergic persons.

ANALGESIC   A drug, such as aspirin or ibuprofen, that reduces pain.

ANAPHYLAXIS   A severe and exceedingly dangerous allergic reaction, characterized by light-headedness, vomiting, cramps, and swollen throat passages that make breathing difficult. Suffocation and death may follow if the reaction is not treated immediately.

ANGIOEDEMA   Giant hives usually accompanied by swelling.

ANTIBODY   A protein molecule the body produces to fight off foreign substances.

ANTIGEN   Any substance, including toxins, viruses, bacteria, and chemicals, that the body perceives as an invader and that induces antibody formation. Used interchangeably with "allergen." (For the sake of clarity, this book uses only "aller-gen.")

ANTIHISTAMINE   A medication that dries mucus and blocks the effects of histamine, a chemical manufactured by certain body cells; used to prevent or stop allergic reactions.

ARTHRALGIA   Pain in a joint.

ASTHMA   A condition, usually allergic, caused by obstructed bronchial tubes. Symptoms include coughing, wheezing, shortness of breath, and chest constriction.

ATOPY   An inherited tendency to produce IgE antibodies to allergens.

AUTOIMMUNE   A condition wherein the body makes antibodies against its own tissue or fluids.

AVOIDANCE   The best way to treat allergies, by clearing away or staying away from known or suspected allergens.

BETA-BLOCKERS   Drugs usually used for high blood pressure and heart disorders; they produce constriction of the airways as a side effect and are usually harmful to asthmatics.

BETA-2 AGONISTS   Drugs that relax bronchial muscles.

BINDER   A substance added to pills or tablets to help hold them together.

BIODEGRADABLE   A common claim on cleaning products, meaning that they are readily decomposed by microorganisms in water, soil, and septic systems.

BIOFEEDBACK   The technique of trying to consciously regulate a body function thought to be involuntary, such as brain waves or heartbeat.

BRONCHI   (Singular: bronchus). The two main branches of the trachea leading to the lungs. Also called bronchial tubes.

BRONCHITIS   Inflammation of the mucous membrane of the bronchial tubes.

BRONCHODILATOR   A medicine that opens the airways.

BRONCHOSPASM   A narrowing or constriction of the airways.

CANDIDA ALBICANS   A genus of yeastlike fungi normally

found in the body, but which can multiply and possibly cause infections, toxicity, or allergic sensitivity.

CANDIDIASIS   Yeast disease; an infection caused by an overgrowth of the yeastlike fungi that are part of the normal flora of the mouth, skin, intestinal tract, and vagina.

CARCINOGEN   Any subject or agent that tends to produce a cancer.

CENTRAL NERVOUS SYSTEM   The brain and spinal cord serving as a command module governing networks of nerves.

CEREBRAL ALLERGY   Mental dysfunction caused by sensitivity to foods, chemicals, inhalants, or irritants in the environment.

CHALLENGE TESTING   A method of determining sensitivity by touching, eating, or inhaling a suspected substance and watching for a reaction.

CHRONIC   Describing a recurrent disease or one of long duration.

CLINICAL   Having to do with the treatment of ill people as opposed to experiments with laboratory animals.

CLINICAL ECOLOGY   Environmental medicine; a branch of medicine that treats both classic and environmental allergies with diet, immunotherapy, and environmental control, and preferably without the use of drugs.

COLONIC IRRIGATION   A highly controversial treatment that involves giving an enema to rid the body of toxins.

CONJUNCTIVITIS   An inflammation of the conjunctiva, the mucous membrane that lines the inner eyelid.

CONTACTANT   A substance that touches the skin.

CONTACT DERMATITIS   A skin rash resulting from touching or rubbing some material.

CORTICOSTEROIDS (CCS)   A family of potent hormones used therapeutically to treat inflammatory and allergic diseases; can be produced naturally in the adrenal glands or synthesized in a laboratory.

CORTISONE   A corticosteroid (produced in the adrenal gland or in a laboratory) that helps regulate the immune system.

CROMOLYN   Cromolyn sodium; a drug used to stabilize mast cells and prevent an allergic reaction.

CROUP   A viral infection that causes hoarseness and breathing difficulties in children.

CUMULATIVE REACTION   A reaction caused by an accumulation of allergens in the body.

CYTOTOXIC TEST   A blood test purporting to determine food and chemical allergies by noting the action of an antigen on the patient's white blood cells.

DANDER   Tiny particles of skin or hair of an animal, which frequently cause allergies.

DECONGESTANT   A drug that shrinks swollen membranes and blood vessels, especially in the sinuses.

DERMATITIS   Inflammation of the skin due to any of many causes. (See *contact dermatitis*.)

DERMOGRAPHISM   Appearance of hives or red welts on the skin as a result of stroking, rubbing, or pressure.

DESENSITIZATION   A process to reduce allergy by injecting gradually increasing amounts of the offending allergen. A more accurate terms is *hyposensitization*, because complete desensitization is never achieved. (See *immunotherapy*.)

DETOXIFICATION   The process of removing or neutralizing toxic substances in the body.

DIGESTIVE SYSTEM   A group of organs, including the mouth,

stomach, liver, pancreas, and intestines, that changes food into forms the body can absorb or excrete.

DOUBLE-BLIND TRIAL   A controlled study of a drug in a clinical situation in which neither the administrators nor the recipients know which patients are getting an active substance and which are receiving a placebo.

ECZEMA   A dry, itchy, noncontagious skin rash usually caused by allergy.

EDEMA   Swelling of body tissue due to excessive fluid.

ELIMINATION DIET   A diet that temporarily eliminates commonly allergenic foods and those suspected of causing allergic symptoms in a specific patient.

EMPHYSEMA   A chronic lung disease.

ENDORPHINS   Morphine-like chemicals produced by the brain and released after strenuous exercise; said to relieve pain and induce feelings of euphoria and well-being.

ENVIRONMENT   The total circumstances or surroundings in which an organism exists.

ENVIRONMENTAL ILLNESS   A complex set of symptoms caused by adverse reactions to substances in the environment.

ENZYME   A substance, usually a protein formed in living cells, that starts or stops biochemical reactions.

EOSINOPHIL   A type of white blood cell that, in increased numbers, indicates the presence of allergy or parasitic infection.

EPINEPHRINE   A powerful adrenal hormone that prepares the body for "fight or flight" by stimulating the heart, raising blood pressure, and constricting blood vessels. It also relaxes bronchial spasms and is vital to treating anaphylactic shock. Trade name: Adrenalin.

EXTRACT   The treatment dilution of an allergen used in testing and immunotherapy.

FDA   The Food and Drug Administration, a government regulatory agency.

FOOD FAMILY   A grouping of foods with similar botanical or biological characteristics.

FORMALDEHYDE   A colorless, irritating gas used chiefly as a disinfectant and preservative.

FRAGRANCE   Any natural or synthetic substance used solely to impart an odor to a cosmetic product.

FRAGRANCE-FREE   A frequently misleading term that suggests a product may be nonirritating or nonallergenic.

FUNGUS   Any of a large group of lower parasitic plants lacking chlorophyll, including molds, yeasts, mildews, and mushrooms.

GAMETE   A male or female reproductive cell.

GASTROINTESTINAL   Pertaining to the digestive tract, including the esophagus, stomach, small intestine, large intestine, and rectum.

GENERIC   The name of a drug as distinct from the registered brand name of the same chemical preparation.

GENETIC   Inherited through the parents' genes.

GENITOURINARY   Genital plus urinary; the body's reproductive and urinary system, including kidneys, urethra, bladder, and genitals.

GLUCOSE   A simple sugar that is easily absorbed into body metabolism.

GLUTEN   A protein in wheat and other grains thought to produce an allergic reaction (usually cramps and diarrhea) in susceptible people.

HERBALISM   The practice of treating illness with herb medication.

HISTAMINE   An organic compound released in allergic reactions, which causes dilation of capillaries, constriction of the bronchi, and increased gastric secretion.

HOLISTIC   An approach to medicine that treats the person as a whole and focuses on nutrition, living habits, and a positive emotional outlook.

HOMEOPATHY   A method of treating disease based on the theory that a substance that produces disease in a healthy person will also, in minute doses, cure the disease.

HORMONE   A chemical substance, secreted by a gland, that travels through the blood to another part of the body where it exerts its stimulatory effect.

HYDRATION   Combining with water.

HYPER-   A prefix meaning more than normal.

HYPERSENSITIVITY   The allergic state.

HYPERSOMNIA   Excessive sleep or drowsiness.

HYPO-   A prefix meaning less than normal.

HYPOALLERGENIC   Products formulated to contain fewer allergens and be less likely to cause allergic reactions. Such products are not necessarily safe for everyone.

IGE   Immunoglobulin E, an antibody specific to allergy.

IGG   Immunoglobulin G, a blocking antibody that prevents IgE from releasing histamine.

IMMUNE RESPONSE   The body's natural reaction to foreign substances.

IMMUNE SYSTEM   The body's mechanism for resisting disease by producing antibodies to neutralize, metabolize, or eliminate antigens.

IMMUNITY   Inherited, acquired, or induced resistance to infection. The state of being able to resist a particular antigen by producing antibodies to counteract it.

IMMUNODEFICIENCY   A loss of some or all of the immune system functions.

IMMUNOGLOBULIN   A specific antibody. See *IgE* and *IgG*.

IMMUNOTHERAPY   The process of building up the body's tolerance to a substance by repeated exposure to the diluted allergen.

IMMUNOTOXIC   Pertaining to chemicals that do the greatest harm to the immune system.

INERT   Without physiological action, as a placebo.

INFECTION   Invasion of the body by a harmful microorganism; also, the disease caused by the invasion.

INFLAMMATION   The body's response to injury, irritants, or infection with pain, heat, reddening, and swelling.

INGESTANT   Anything swallowed or taken by mouth.

INHALANT   Any airborne substance such as pollen or mold spores tiny enough to be inhaled into the lungs.

INHALER or METERED DOSE INHALER   An aerosol device used to administer medicine while the patient breathes in.

INTRADERMAL TEST   An allergy test performed by injecting antigen beneath the outer layer of the skin and measuring the wheal it provokes.

IN VITRO   Literally, "in glass." In vitro tests do not involve living vertebrate animals.

IN VIVO   Literally, "in life" or "on the living body," as in skin tests.

IRRITANT   Any substance that causes (usually) local inflammation.

LACTATE   To secrete milk.

LACTASE   An intestinal enzyme that converts lactose into more digestible glucose and galactose.

LACTOSE   A sugar derived from milk.

MAST CELLS   Large cells containing histamine found in the mucous membranes, bronchial tubes, and skin.

MICROORGANISMS   Living creatures too small to be seen with the naked eye; also known as germs. They include bacteria, fungi, and viruses.

MIGRAINE   A severe vascular headache, often accompanied by nausea and vomiting and preceded by visual disturbances; frequently attributed to food allergy.

MUCOUS MEMBRANE   The body's inside skin; soft layers of cells that line the surface of certain body tracts such as the respiratory and gastrointestinal.

MUCUS   The thick liquid secreted by the mucous membranes to protect openings in the body.

MYALGIA   Muscle pain or soreness.

NASAL POLYPS   Fluid-filled growths in the nose that frequently block the nasal passages and are sometimes related to allergies.

NEBULIZER   An apparatus that delivers medication through the mouth as a fine mist or spray.

NEUTRALIZE   To render an allergic reaction inactive.

NYSTATIN   One of several antifungal antibiotics that selectively attacks *Candida albicans*.

OPTIMAL DOSE   Dose that gives the most relief for the longest period of time.

ORGANIC   Pertaining to foods grown in soil free of chemical fertilizers, pesticides, fungicides, and herbicides.

OSHA   Occupational Safety and Health Administration, a federal government agency.

OUTGAS   The release of volatile chemicals that evaporate slowly and continuously from seemingly stable materials such as polyester, plastic, and building materials.

OVER-THE-COUNTER (OTC) DRUG   A drug that the FDA has approved as safe for self-medication, available without a prescription.

PARASITE   An organism that depends on a host organism for food and shelter and contributes nothing to the host.

PEAK EXPIRATORY FLOW RATE   The maximum rate at which air can be exhaled.

PEAK-FLOW METER   A device used to measure peak expiratory flow and predict an asthma attack.

PETROCHEMICAL   A synthetic chemical derived from petroleum or natural gas.

PHOTOPHOBIA   Abnormal visual intolerance to light.

PHOTOSENSITIVITY   Abnormal sensitivity of the skin to ultraviolet light, usually following exposure to drugs or other sensitizing chemicals.

PLACEBO   A medically inert subject formulated to resemble an active substance, used to test the efficacy of that substance.

POLLEN   The microscopic seeds of trees, grasses, and flowers that form a fine, airborne dust and can cause allergic reactions.

POLLUTANT   Any gaseous, chemical, or organic substance that contaminates air, water, or the physical body.

POSTNASAL DRIP   A condition in which nasal fluids leak down into the back of the pharynx, often causing a sore throat.

PROVOCATIVE-NEUTRALIZATION (P-N) TEST   An allergy test that uses an allergen to provoke a reaction, then attempts to neutralize the reaction with a lower or higher dose of the same allergen that produced it.

PSYCHOSOMATIC   Referring to an ailment or group of ailments known to be caused by emotional factors.

PSYCHOTHERAPY   The treatment of emotional disorders primarily by interaction between patient (or groups of patients) and therapist.

PULMONARY   Pertaining to the lungs.

RADIOALLERGOSORBENT TEST (RAST)   A blood test to measure IgE in the blood and determine allergies.

REBOUND EFFECT   A severe flare-up of symptoms that occurs when medicine is suddenly withdrawn.

RESPIRATORY TRACT   The system that starts at the nostrils, runs through the nose to the back of the throat, then down into the larynx and lungs.

RHINITIS   Inflammation of the mucous membrane of the nose; a nasal condition characterized by sneezing, congestion, and a watery discharge.

ROTATION DIET   A diet in which particular foods are eaten only once every four to seven days.

SALICYLATES   A class of compounds of which aspirin is the best known, used to reduce pain, inflammation, and body temperature.

SENSITIZATION   The initial exposure of an individual to a specific antigen, resulting in an immune response; subsequent exposure then producing a much stronger response.

SHOCK ORGAN or TARGET ORGAN   The organ or system of a person most affected by a particular allergy.

SINUSITIS   Bacterial infection of the sinus cavities.

SKIN TEST   A test for allergy done by scratching or pricking the skin, applying a suspected allergen, and measuring the reaction.

SMEAR   A sample of blood, mucus, or other body material spread on a glass slide for examination under a microscope.

SOLVENT   A substance, usually liquid, that can dissolve another substance.

SPACER   An apparatus inserted between the mouth and an inhaler to increase the amount of medication reaching the lungs.

SPIROMETER   A device used to measure air volume in the lungs.

SPORE   A single cell of a simple organism, such as fungus, that becomes detached from the parent and reproduces.

SPUTUM   Mucus, sometimes mixed with pus, coughed up from the lungs; phlegm.

STEROID   A synthetic compound used to suppress the action of the immune system.

STRESS   Anything that places undue strain on normal body functions. It can be internal, due to allergy or disease, or external, due to personal relations or environmental factors.

SUBLINGUAL   Under the tongue; a method of testing or treating allergens that involves rapid absorption.

SYMPTOM   The body's signal to you that something is wrong.

SYNDROME   A set of symptoms that characterize a specific disease or disorder.

SYNTHETIC   Man-made; not produced normally in nature.

SYSTEMIC   Pertaining to the whole body rather than to one of its parts, as in a systemic reaction.

TARGET ORGAN   The organ or system of a person most affected by a particular allergy. Same as shock organ.

THEOPHYLLINE   A bronchodilator, chemically related to caffeine.

THERAPY   Any form of medical treatment.

TOLERANCE THRESHOLD   The maximum amount of allergens a person can endure without reacting.

TOPICAL   Affecting only one location or organ.

TOXIC   Poisonous. Effects range from harmful to lethal depending on dose taken and resistance of the individual.

TOXIN   Any poisonous or irritating substance.

TRANSFER FACTOR   An extract of white blood cells said to transfer immunity from donor to recipient.

TYRAMINE   An organic substance found in certain foods that is capable of swelling blood cells and is said to provoke migraines.

URINARY SYSTEM   The kidneys, ureter, bladder, and urethra; organs involved in the filtration of toxins and the secretion and discharge of urine.

URTICARIA   Allergic hives or welts.

URUSHIOL   The irritating oil in the sap of poison oak and poison ivy that causes an itchy skin rash.

VASCULAR   Pertaining to blood vessels.

WHEAL   A sudden elevation of the skin surface that is measured to determine the degree of allergic sensitivity.

WHEEZING   A hissing, whistling sound caused by difficulty breathing.

WITHDRAWAL   The psychic and physiological adjustment to discontinuing a habit or use of a habit-forming substance.

INDEX